TCRN®
STUDY GUIDE

Trauma Certified Registered Nurse

Pamela D. Bartley, BSN, RN, CEN, TCRN, CCRN, CFRN, CTRN, CPEN
PDB Nurse Education, LLC

TCRN Study Guide

PDB Nurse Education, LLC **Study and Test Taking Tips**

- Check www.BCEN.org for exam information, live remote proctoring option, purchasing **vouchers** to reduce exam fee, sample questions, and **FAQ**'s.
- Take the current edition of **TNCC (9th edition), ATCN, or TCAR**. Live and virtual TNCC courses can be found on the ENA website under the Education University. My sample questions and posttest, and critical thinking questions are referenced to **TNCC 9th edition, 2023**.
- Download and read the **FREE** download American College of Surgeons *Optimal Care of the Injured Patient*.
- **Register for the exam ASAP**, it makes it "real", and you will actively study. Schedule your exam at the **best time of the day for you**, morning, or afternoon. **Do not tell anyone your test date**, it just adds more pressure.
- The **TCRN exam is 175 questions**, you have **180 minutes** to complete the exam. All questions are multiple-choice, there are no "all of the above" or 'select all that apply". Twenty-five questions are NOT graded, and the passing score is **104/150**. The **2022 TCRN pass rate was 58%**.
- Plan as if you are preparing for a marathon, schedule study time! Prepare a **dedicated study space**, have flashcards or a notebook to write content you need to learn more when studying the **"Physiology Review"**. Study during your peak brain time, in 30-45-minute intervals. Study the **"Sample Questions"** and rationales. Take the 60-question "**Posttest**" in 60 minutes and ensure you score 75% or higher. Assess your content knowledge through the **"Critical Thinking."**
- **Do not cram** the night before, you do not test as well when your brain is tired. Get a good night's **sleep and eat** a healthy breakfast/lunch prior to exam, but do not overhydrate.
- Approach exam with CONFIDENCE! Visualize the win! Control your anxiety, **practice deep breathing and visualization**. Ignore self-defeating thoughts.
- Read each question carefully and ask yourself, **"What is the question really asking?"** looking for "**key words**" like **priority**, initial intervention, first, earliest, least likely, or best.
- Do NOT read into the question. All information needed is in the scenario (take it at face value). Do NOT be misled by **"close-to-correct"** answers that often precede the correct answer.
- Be alert to questions that say INCORRECT, **EXCEPT**, NOT correct. Read the four choices for which answer **does not fit**. Do NOT be taken in by unfamiliar words.
- Do NOT assume an answer is correct because you have observed the action in your nursing practice. Let **evidence-based practice** guide your response.
- When in doubt, go with your **first response** and **do NOT change answers unless you misinterpreted the question**. Do **NOT get immobilized** by a question! Answer it the best you can and move on. Let it go!
- Pam says, **"You Can Do It**!" You get your score as soon as you complete the exam. Email me at pbartleysc@gmail.com after you ace the exam!

PDB Nurse Education, LLC TCRN Trauma Physiology Review

Head and Neck Trauma – 33 questions

1. ABC's - airway first (suctioning)/alertness, breathing, and circulation are priorities unless massive hemorrhage on across-the-room. Treat the greatest life-threatening condition first.
2. Glasgow Coma Scale (GCS) evaluates best eye opening, best verbal response, and best motor response. Airway protection is the priority if GCS 8 or less. FOUR score evaluates eye, motor, brain reflexes, and respiration, so better to use in intubated patients. Review AVPU – alert, response to voice, response to pain, unresponsive.
3. Stabilize penetrating objects.
4. Monroe-Kellie doctrine = volume-pressure relationship of skull.
    a. Normal ICP for adults is 3-15 mmHg. Infants – 2-6, young – 3-7, older child 10-15.
    b. Increased ICP if sustained > 20-22 mmHg. ICP peaks 48-72 hours post injury.
    c. Cerebral perfusion pressure (CPP) = MAP-ICP (normal 60-100, texts differ on exact number); keep > 60 mmHg in TBI.
5. Cerebral spinal fluid (CSF) leakage – do not pack, apply a sterile dressing under nose (nasal drip pad) to allow free drainage, but avoid infection.
6. Early **S/S of increased ICP** include nausea and vomiting and headache. Late S/S include Cushing's Triad - widened pulse pressure (increasing SBP), bradycardia, and decreased respiratory effort (ataxic respirations possible). Suspect spinal cord injury (SCI) if patient bradycardic, but hypotensive (neurogenic shock).
7. **Basilar skull fracture (BSF)**
    a. Anterior fossa fracture - rhinorrhea, periorbital ecchymosis "Raccoon's eyes", and anosmia (CNI).
    b. Middle fossa fracture – otorrhea, mastoid ecchymosis "Battle's Sign", hemotympanum.
    c. Assess glucose if clear drainage, see halo sign if bloody.
8. **Epidural hematoma (EDH)**
    a. Middle meningeal artery tear from temporal bone injury.
    b. Rapid onset – classic S/S - unresponsive, lucid period, second unresponsiveness.
    c. Uncal herniation – ipsilateral pupil dilation, contralateral hemiparesis.
    d. Burr holes for emergency treatment since blood above the dura; reverse anticoagulants.
9. **Subdural hematoma (SDH)**
    a. Tear of the venous bridging veins.
    b. Slower decompensation of mental status, "not acting right"; progresses over hours to weeks.
    c. More often in elderly, and alcoholics due to frequent falls.
    d. Shaken impact syndrome – triad of SDH, retinal hemorrhage, and posterior rib fractures. Notify child protective services ASAP and keep child safe.
10. **Concussion**
    a. PECARN criteria for head CT in pediatrics – Get CT if GCS < 15, altered LOC, not acting normally.
    b. Cognitive rest so do not wake up frequently, no caffeine to stimulate brain.
    c. No aspirin or NSAIDs due to risk of bleed, acetaminophen only for pain, no narcotics
    d. Medically clearance by concussion specialist, graduated return to play. No school until symptoms resolved. May have post-concussive syndrome.
    e. Risk of secondary impact syndrome which may cause death.
11. **Diffuse Axonal Injury**
    a. S/S: Hyperthermia, HTN, profuse sweating, deep prolonged coma, abnormal posturing.
    b. TX: Management of increased ICP, monitor for diabetes insipidus (DI) due to pressure on posterior pituitary decreasing ADH, leading to polyuria. Treat DI with vasopressin (ADH).
12. **Management of increased intracranial pressure (ICP)** – Spikes 48-72 hours post injury.
    a. Hypertonic saline preferred if hypotensive, then loop diuretics (Lasix) or osmotic diuretics.
    b. Mannitol (osmotic diuretic) bolus if hemodynamically stable. Reduces ICP within 1-5 minutes, peaks at 20-60 minutes. Monitor for pulmonary edema initially.
        i. Monitor potassium, sodium, and serum osmolality (keep at 300-320 mOsm).
    c. Keep SBP > 100 -100 mmHg, no permissive hypotension allowed in head injury.
    d. Keep CO_2 at 35-37 and avoid hypoxemia (keep O2 sat > 95%) to prevent secondary brain injury.
    e. Transfuse if hemoglobin low to increase oxygen-carrying capacity.

f. Reverse anticoagulants – Kcentra and vitamin K if patient on warfarin (Coumadin), or Andexxa if patient is on Xarelto or Eliquis.
g. Elevate HOB to 30-45 degrees, head in neutral alignment, remove rigid cervical collar.
h. Quiet and dark environment, limit visitors, speak softly, treat anxiety and pain (Fentanyl decreases ICP, may use Propofol if frequent assessments are needed), no music initially, treat fever aggressively.

13. Early interventions to avoid long-term complications of traumatic brain injury (TBI).
    a. Feed early, nutrition to reduce stress ulcers and sepsis, helps with wound healing.
    b. DVT prophylaxis through compression, and early mobilization with physical therapy. Turn often to reduce skin breakdown.
    c. Treat hyperglycemia, keep glucose 80-120 mg/dl.

14. **Ocular emergencies**
    a. Corneal abrasion – do not patch eyes, increases risk of infection.
    b. Alkaline (ammonia, lye, drain cleaner, cement) ocular burns worse than acids. Irrigate immediately with warmed LR/NS (37 degrees C), until pH 7.4
    c. Ruptured globe – tear-dropped shaped pupil, secure impaled object with cup. Do NOT instill eye drops, further protrudes intraocular contents.. Shield eye with a rigid shield, not pressure dressing.
    d. Orbital wall fracture - pain and limited upward gaze on EOM assessment, pressure on CN III (oculomotor). Look for associated ocular injuries such as ruptured globe.
    e. Hyphema – blood in anterior chamber, reddish hue to vision. Keep patient upright 30-45 degrees for 3-5 days, but do not lean forward since it increases IOP, and no reading. The highest rebleed risk is in 3-5 days.
    f. Retrobulbar hematoma – administer mannitol and prepare to perform a lateral canthotomy.

15. **Facial injuries**
    a. Use caution when using xylocaine with epinephrine ear and nose since decreased blood flow at end-arterial points due to risk of infection.
    b. Mandibular fracture – malocclusion and lower lip/jaw paresthesia; airway occlusion from loss of tongue control.
    c. Zygomatic – loss of malar eminence (cheekbone prominence).
    d. Le Fort maxillary fractures – priority is maintenance of airway, keep in high-fowlers, tonsil-tip suction. Do not insert NG tube.
        i. I – free-floating maxilla, lip laceration
        ii. II – pyramidal-shaped fracture, nasal fracture
        iii. III – craniofacial separation, severe swelling, decreased LOC.

16. **Neck injuries**
    a. Check c-spine. Direct pressure initially while monitoring airway.
    b. Strangulation – stroke-like symptoms from blood clots, red flag in interpersonal violence.
    c. Most neck injuries are in zone II, zone I injuries most lethal due to blood vessels and lungs. Cranial nerve IX glossopharyngeal dysfunction results in difficulty swallowing.
    d. Tracheobronchial and laryngeal injury- clothesline type injury (all-terrain vehicle or dirt-bike rider into suspended cable) or penetrating injury.
        i. S/S: Hamman's sign (crunch with heartbeat) and SQ emphysema, stridor, increasing hematoma = respiratory distress. Continuous bubbling in chest drainage system.
        ii. Laryngeal (voice box) injury – dysphonia (voice change, hoarseness)
        iii. TX: Fiberoptic intubation or emergency repair.
    e. Esophageal injury – food particles in chest drainage system and subcutaneous emphysema.

17. **Spinal cord injury (SCI)**
    a. Increased risk of SCI if fall > 20 feet in adult, > 2-3 times child's height (approx.. > 10 feet).
    b. Log rolling can cause secondary injuries including SCI and hemorrhage from pelvic fractures. Lift and slide preferred.
    c. Guide cervical spine clearance and radiologic exam need.
        i. Canadian C-spine rule – dangerous MOI, age > 65, neck rotation, numbness/tingling. "Sixty-five, fast drive, sense deprive? Image, of alive." "Slow wreck, slow neck, sitting down and walking around? C-spine fine."
        ii. NEXUS criteria – NSAID mnemonic - midline cervical **N**eck tenderness, focal neuro **S**ensory deficit, **A**lertness, **I**ntoxication, painful **D**istracting injury.

d. Spinal motion restriction – rigid cervical collar and keeping head, neck, and torso in alignment. Spine boards, scoop stretcher, vacuum mattress for transfer only.
e. Chance lumbar fracture (lap belt injury) is associated with hollow organ injury (bowel, stomach).
f. Suspect SCI if absent bowel sounds without abdominal injury, plus bradycardia and hypotension.
g. SCIWORA (without radiographic abnormality) in child < age 8 – get MRI to see edema.
h. Paralysis - High-cervical C1-C4 – focus on airway and breathing (C3, 4, 5 keeps your diaphragm alive). C5-C8 – some control of arms and hands (C 5, 6, 7 – raise arms to heaven). T1-T5 (paraplegia). L1-L5 – may walk with braces. S1-S5 – most able to walk, but little control of bowel and bladder.
i. Complete spinal cord injury – Priapism, poikilothermia, loss of bowel and bladder function. Monitor skin early, DVT prophylaxis. Monitor and treat neurogenic shock.
j. Neurogenic shock
   i. Distributive shock – low systemic vascular resistance (SVR afterload) due to vasodilation.
   ii. Neurogenic shock is the only type of shock with bradycardia initially.
   iii. Loss of sympathetic nervous system innervation, leaving unopposed parasympathetic that slows down.
   iv. S/S: bradycardia (or lack of expected tachycardia), bradypnea, poikilothermia (hypothermia), priapism, anhydrosis (no sweating), and hypotension.
   v. TX: Augment vascular tone with fluids, Norepinephrine, and Dopamine.
   vi. Spinal shock – transient flaccidity and loss of reflexes.
k. **Incomplete cord injury** – patient has sacral sparing (voluntary anal sphincter tone).
   i. Anterior cord syndrome – most common, motor loss; spares vibration and proprioception. Requires extensive rehabilitation since motor loss.
   ii. Central cord syndrome – increased deficit in upper extremities versus lower extremities, seen in older patients; requires extensive rehabilitation.
   iii. Brown-Sequard syndrome – ipsilateral motor function loss with contralateral loss of sensation, mostly from penetrating injury.

Trunk Trauma - 37 questions

Thoracic Trauma

1. Leave impaled object in place and stabilize since the object tamponades the bleed.
2. FAST exam evaluates pericardium, hepatorenal, splenorenal, and pelvis (life-threatening).
3. **Rib fractures** – painful, so goal is pain control with NSAIDs, lidocaine transdermal, epidural, On-Q pump, operative fixation.
   a. 1st and 2nd – great vessel injury of aorta at ligamentum arteriosum. Get an arteriogram for diagnosis.
   b. 4-9 ribs (most common) – pulmonary contusion common, so decrease IVF infusion rate.
   c. Right lower rib fractures – suspect liver injury. Left lower rib fractures – suspect splenic injury.
   d. Posterior rib fractures – suspect renal injury.
4. **Aortic dissection** – aorta shears at ligamentum arteriosum, mostly from blunt trauma.
   a. S/S: Bilateral blood pressure differences, decreased pulses in lower extremities, new onset murmur, widened mediastinum and obscured aortic knob on x-ray.
   b. TX: surgical repair, massive transfusion protocol, beta-blockers to keep HR 60-80 and SBP 100-120 mm Hg.
5. **Pulmonary contusion** – S/S: wheezing and crackles, most common 24-48 hours after insult. Risk of acute respiratory distress syndrome (ARDS), so judicious use of IVFs to achieve euvolemia; keep SpO_2 94-98%.
6. **ARDS** – refractory hypoxemia, P:F ratio < 200, "white out" on x-ray 48-72 hours after insult. TX: recruit alveoli with lower tidal volumes (6 ml/kg) and 10-15 mm Hg of PEEP to decrease shunting, prone positioning, and high-frequency ventilation.
7. **Pulmonary embolism** (PE) – sudden onset of restlessness, respiratory distress, and hypoxemia. CT pulmonary angiography is the gold standard for diagnosis. Prevent PE by avoiding venous stasis (early ambulation, compression) and monitoring for DVT.
8. **Flail chest** – paradoxical chest wall movement due to two or more rib fractures at two or more places, monitor respiration, early intubation, immediate fixation required, concurrent pulmonary contusion so decrease IVF administration.

9. **Pneumothorax** (air-leak syndrome)
    a. S/S: Decreased to absent breath sounds on affected side, hyperresonance on percussion.
    b. Positive-pressure ventilation can worsen a pneumothorax.
    c. **Open pneumothorax**
        i. S/S: Sucking chest wound on inhalation, bubbling blood on exhalation.
        ii. TX: Oxygen, occlusive dressing secured at 3-sides at end-exhalation temporarily or use a flutter valve. Remove the dressing if the patient has signs of increased respiratory distress (possible tension pneumothorax).
    d. **Tension pneumothorax** – most life-threatening pneumothorax (obstructive shock, risk of PEA)
        i. S/S: Respiratory distress, JVD, hypotension increased inspiration, absent or reduced breath sounds on affected side, tracheal deviation to unaffected side.
        ii. TX: Needle thoracostomy/decompression immediately 2nd ICS mid-clavicular line or 5th ICS anterior axillary line.
10. **Hemothorax** – prepare for chest tube and consider autotransfusion if blunt trauma. Notify trauma if > 1500 ml immediately or > 200 mL per hour for 2-4 hours.
    a. Advantages of autotransfusion – warm, readily available, no transfusion reaction, decreased risk of communicable disease, lower potassium level, better oxygen-carrying capacity. Risk of contamination in penetrating injury.
11. **Chest drainage systems** – tape all connections, keep upright below the level of the chest, coil the tubing without dependent loops or kinks. Assess for FOCA – Fluctuations, Output, Color, Air leak, and bubbling.
    a. Tidaling in water-seal chamber is normal with respiration.
    b. Continuous bubbling is a sign of an air leak.
    c. Clamping chest tube may cause a tension pneumothorax.
12. **Blunt cardiac injury** (cardiac contusion) may be associated with fractured sternum, the right ventricle is most often damaged. ECG: ST segment elevation, sinus tachycardia, premature ventricular contractions, and hypotension; requires continuous cardiac monitoring and repeat echocardiograms, monitor for cardiogenic shock.
13. **Pericardial tamponade** (obstructive shock)
    a. S/S: Becks triad = JVD, hypotension, and muffled (distant) heart sounds. Also see tachycardia, anxiousness, restlessness, electrical alternans or low ECG voltage, and pulsus paradoxus.
    b. DX: FAST exam. TX: Resuscitative thoracotomy or surgical pericardiectomy to make a "window", especially effective for penetrating injury. Needle pericardiocentesis is temporary fix.
14. **Resuscitative Endovascular Balloon Occlusion of the Aorta - REBOA** – Insertion into femoral artery into the descending aorta, Zone 1 for traumatic arrest.
15. **Airway management**
    a. Nasopharyngeal airways (NPA) are contraindicated in basilar skull fractures and facial trauma since the NPA may go through the cribriform plate into cranial vault.
    b. The purpose of **drug-assisted intubation** is to decrease the risk of aspiration.
        i. Administer a sedative such as etomidate prior to the neuromuscular blocking agent to avoid tachycardia and increased ICP from patient experiencing pain.
        ii. Place the bed in reverse trendelenburg position at 30 degrees.
        iii. Succinylcholine is contraindicated with family history of malignant hyperthermia, rhabdomyolysis, myasthenia gravis. Consider Rocuronium instead.
    c. Auscultate over the epigastrium first after endotracheal intubation, then for bilateral breath sounds.
    d. Auscultate breath sounds axillary in children since breath sounds transmit across the chest.
    e. Administer one breath every 6 seconds (10 breaths/minute. Excessive volume and rates cause gastric distention, which leads to vomiting and aspiration.
    f. Use cuffed ET tubes in pediatrics since frequent transport and higher accuracy of $ETCO_2$.
    g. Normal $ETCO_2$ 35-45 – increase ventilation rate if CO_2 high, decrease ventilation rate if CO_2 low.
    h. Surgical cricothyrotomies are preferred over needle in adults and children over age 12.
    i. **DOPE** mnemonic – Displacement, Obstruction, Pneumothorax, Equipment problems. High pressure alarms from kinked tube, bronchospasm, obstruction from secretions (suction), intra-abdominal compartment pressure.

j. Oxyhemoglobin Dissociation Curve
    i. Left shift – hemoglobin to hold onto oxygen. Increased pH (alkalosis), decreased CO_2, hypothermia, CO poisoning.
    ii. Right shift– body does right thing and delivers more oxygen to cells. Decreased pH (acidosis), increased CO_2, hyperthermia.

16. **Obstetric emergencies**
    a. Resting heart rate increases 10-20 beats/minute. Pregnancy causes an increased risk of aspiration, dilutional anemia, and DIC from HELLP (hemolysis, elevated liver enzymes, low platelets) syndrome.
    b. Pregnant women are twice as likely to experience violence as nonpregnant women. High lap belt may cause uterine rupture.
    c. No pelvic exam until ultrasound if vaginal bleeding.
    d. Turn the patient on their left side to avoid supine vena cava syndrome which decreases venous return to the heart leading to low cardiac output.
    e. Fundal height at umbilicus at 20 weeks gestation, viable fetus (20-24 weeks), 1 cm above = 1 week, EX: 26 cm = 26 weeks pregnant.
    f. Normal fetal heart tones (FHT) are 120-160 bpm, fetal tachycardia is the first sign of distress. Late decelerations are an ominous sign of fetal distress.
    g. Get a Kleihauer-Betke (KB) test to determine fetal cells in maternal blood. Administer Rhogam within 72 hours if mother is Rh negative.
    h. Preterm labor – fetal monitoring, administer tocolytic like magnesium sulfate to halt labor. Administer betamethasone for fetal lung maturation.
    i. Imminent delivery – check for umbilical cord pulsation. Nitrazine paper blue from pH 7.0-7.5 – amniotic fluid from ruptured membranes. Control delivery to reduce perineal tears.
    j. Uterine rupture – increased risk if prior C-sections, sharp abdominal pain, hemorrhagic shock, palpable fetal parts, slowing or absent FHT. TX: immediate c-section and hysterectomy.
    k. Abruptio placentae - ripping abdominal/back pain, board like uterus, rising fundal height, with scant amount of dark red bleeding. TX: immediate C-section. Risk of HELLP syndrome (DIC).
    l. Maternal cardiopulmonary arrest – prepare for C-section, manually displace the uterus to the left to minimize aortocaval compression, perform CPR, defibrillate as needed.
    m. Still apply pelvic binder if open book pelvic fracture, fetus dies if mother bleeds out.

17. **Abdominal trauma**
    a. Palpate the abdominal quadrant opposite of painful area first. FAST exam is diagnostic exam of choice.
    b. Abdominal evisceration – cover with sterile dressing and prepare for surgery. Bloody NG aspirate – suspect injury to the stomach.
    c. Stab wound – injury to LUQ more common since most are right-handed. The small and large bowels are the most injured abdominal organs.
    d. **Ruptured diaphragm** – penetrating injury below the 4th ICS, peristaltic gurgling sounds in left chest, progressively scaphoid abdomen. Kehr's sign (left shoulder pain) worse when supine. Priority is securing airway and assisting breathing until emergent exploratory laparotomy performed.
    e. **Splenic injury**
        i. S/S: LUQ abdominal pain radiating to left shoulder (Kehr's sign) ecchymosis of the left flank.
        ii. Grading – Grade IV - > 25% of spleen injured, Grade V – completely shattered.
        iii. A nonoperative approach preferred to preserve the immunologic function of the spleen.
        iv. Splenectomy – normal to have increased WBC post-op, back to normal by day 4 post-op.
            1. Pneumococcal, meningococcal, influenza vaccines if splenectomy.
    f. **Liver injury**
        i. S/S: RUQ abdominal pain, shock, dullness to percussion, Cullen's sign (ecchymosis around umbilicus).
        ii. DX: Elevated LFT's. Grading I (hematoma) to VI (vascular avulsion).
        iii. TX: Allow permissive hypotension (70/40) to reduce bleeding (do not pop the clot) and prepare for damage-control surgery (under 90 minutes) to control bleeding.
    g. **Bowel rupture** – Lap restraint injury, associated with Chance fracture (T12-L2); transverse colon often injured. Stomach and bowel injury seen in penetrating injury.
    h. **Pancreatic injury** commonly missed initially, sits retroperitoneal (Grey-Turner's sign), epigastric pain radiating to back. Monitor blood glucose, lipase, amylase, and calcium. Risk of fistula (pseudocysts).

i. **Abdominal compartment syndrome -** obstructive shock.
    i. Highest risk – pregnancy, chronic ascites, morbidly obese, major abdominal surgery, peritonitis.
    ii. Abdominal perfusion pressure (APP) = mean arterial pressure (MAP)- Intraabdominal pressure (IAP).
    iii. Bladder pressure monitoring through urinary bladder catheter monitoring.
        1. Level transducer at symphysis pubis with patient in supine position.
        2. Normal reading 12-15 mmHg, reading > 20 may require immediate decompression.

j. **Renal injury** - hematuria, flank tenderness, ecchymosis over flank, rising BUN and creatinine, monitor urine output.

k. **Bladder injury** – urge to urinate but inability to pass urine, urology consultation and get cystogram. Complication is a chemical peritonitis.

i. **Urethral injury** – common with pelvic fractures. Do not insert a urinary catheter if blood at urinary meatus, may need suprapubic catheter. DX: Retrograde urethrogram. Contrast media may cause pre-renal failure, so check creatinine (normal < 1.2), increase fluids, and monitor urine output.

Extremity and Wound Trauma - 25 questions

1. Irrigate with saline or tap water at low pressure to clean, at high pressure to remove bacteria.
2. Avoid xylocaine with epinephrine on digits, ears, nose, and in avulsion injuries since it causes vasoconstriction, increasing infection risk.
3. Remove vegetative (biologic) matter (thorns, splinters, cactus spines) ASAP since they soak in fluid and swell. Do not soak, more difficult to extract foreign body since it swells. Vegetative material does not show on x-ray, so get CT or MRI to identify.
4. Tetanus found in animal excrement, farm injuries highest risk. Administer tetanus immunoglobulin (TIG) in addition to tetanus toxoid if dirty wound and unsure of vaccine status.
5. Poor wound healing in decreased tissue perfusion, poor nutrition, vascular compromise (smoker, diabetes, coronary artery disease, anemia), medications that slow collagen formation (steroids, phenytoin), advanced age.
6. Avulsions/Degloving – scalp is vascular, excessive bleeding. Apply non-adherent dressing.
7. Contusions/hematomas – greater infection risk since blood is a medium for bacterial growth.
8. **High pressure injection injury** from grease guns, hydraulic guns, and paint guns. Substance travels deep into the fascia. - high priority triage, emergent surgical intervention due to saponification and risk of compartment syndrome.
9. Nerve Assessment
    a. Radial nerve – give “thumbs up” or “hitchhike” sign. Median nerve – thumb to 5th finger, make a fist (trapped in forearm and wrist fractures). Ulnar nerve – fan out fingers.
    b. Femoral nerve – flex hip against resistance, Tibial nerve – push down like pressing on gas pedal, Peroneal nerve – pull foot up.
10. **Fractures**
    a. Splint extremity to immobilize joints above and below.
    b. Open fracture – risk is hemorrhage and infection, typically tib-fib fractures.
    c. Cauda equina syndrome – Fall onto coccyx, saddle anesthesia.
    d. **Fall on an outstretched hand (FOOSH) fractures.**
        i. Monteggia fracture – ulnar shaft fracture with radial head dislocation.
        ii. Galeazzi fracture – distal radial fracture with distal ulnar epiphyseal fracture.
        iii. Colles’s fracture – distal radial fracture.
        iv. Scaphoid – pain at anatomic “snuff box”, splint with thumb in opposition, thumb spica splint.
    e. **Boxer’s fracture** – 5th metacarpal fracture from punching, apply posterior ulnar splint after assessing for “fight bite.”
    f. **Pelvic fracture**
        i. Assess with gentle pressure inward and downward.
        ii. Apply pelvic binder at the level of the greater trochanter.
        iii. Allow permissive hypotension and prepare for massive transfusion protocol (MTP) for hemorrhagic shock from tear of iliac artery.

    iv. Surgery or REBOA at Zone 3 if bleeding not controlled.
    v. Pelvic fractures are commonly associated with bladder and urethral injury.
  g. **Femur fracture** – deformity of upper thigh, shortening and rotation, hemorrhagic shock; apply traction splint for mid-shaft femur fracture to decrease bleeding and pain. High risk for fat emboli.
  h. **Calcaneal fracture** – axial loading pressure from landing feet-first, associated tibial plateau and spine compression fractures.

11. **Dislocations**
    a. Frequent vascular checks and reduction ASAP for all dislocations. Monitor closely while sedated.
    b. Shoulder dislocation may cause brachial plexus injury.
    c. **Hip dislocation** – 90% are posterior dislocations, passenger knee to dashboard. Complications include avascular necrosis of the femoral head and sciatic nerve compression.
    d. **Knee dislocation** – complications include popliteal artery and peroneal nerve injury.
12. **Fat embolism syndrome**
    a. Most within 24-72 hours post long-bone (femur) fracture.
    b. S/S: sudden onset of severe respiratory distress with hypoxia, restlessness to decreased mental status, and petechial rash on chest, axillae, and conjunctivae. Patchy pulmonary infiltrates and ground glass opacities on x-ray.
13. **Gunshot wounds**
    a. Velocity (speed) more important than mass, rifles increase speed.
    b. Hollow point – less likely to exit.
    c. Lower velocity – tumble and yaw, ricochet once inside, surgical intervention.
    d. Shotgun from distance – pellets scatter, potentially causing emboli.
14. **Amputation**
    a. Hemorrhage control of stump is top priority – direct pressure to site, a tourniquet (or 2) to control bleeding.
    b. Tourniquets – place as close to the amputation site as possible. Mark time applied! May need second tourniquet applied 2 inches above first. Must be tight enough to compress veins and arteries. Do not release until surgeon is prepared to manage the bleeding.
    c. Gently rinse the amputated part, wrap in sterile saline-moistened gauze and place in Ziplock bag, place bag on top of second bag of ice. Avoid direct contact with ice.
15. **Crush injury** - risk of compartment syndrome, rhabdomyolysis, and acute kidney injury.
16. **Rhabdomyolysis** – seen in prolonged down time.
    a. Myalgia (muscle pain), dark red or brown urine; elevated CK, myoglobin, and potassium levels. pH low, metabolic acidosis.
    b. TX: IVF's, systemic alkalization with sodium bicarbonate until urine pH > 8.0, mannitol, dialysis, goal is urine output of 100 to 300 ml/hr.
    c. Complication – acute tubular necrosis (acute renal failure)
17. **Compartment syndrome**
    a. S/S: pain out of proportion, unrelieved by analgesia, on passive movement, shiny taut skin; most occur in lower leg (4 compartments) or forearm. Weak or absent pulses are an ominous sign.
    b. Normal pressure 0-10 mmHg, in neutral position (level of heart) if 20 mmHg, no ice, possible fasciotomy if > 30.
18. An **Ankle-Brachial Index** (ABI) is the ratio of pressure in the ankle to brachium. Normal is 0.9-1.2, < 0.9 may help detect occult arterial vascular injuries. May also assess arterial pressure index.
19. **Burns**
    a. Secure airway immediately if hoarse voice, stridor, carbonaceous sputum. Prepare for an escharotomy to relieve external compression and allow chest expansion if advised by burn center.
    b. **Carbon monoxide (CO)**
        i. Toxic > 25%, lethal > 60%, cherry red skin.
        ii. O_2 saturation will be normal since hemoglobin holds onto oxygen (left shift of oxyhemoglobin dissociation curve), ST segment depression from hypoxia.
        iii. TX: 100% oxygen until carboxyhemoglobin is < 10% (approx. 1 hour); pregnant patient may require hyperbaric oxygen (HBO) to get oxygen to fetus.
    c. **Hydrogen Cyanide** – smell of bitter almonds, antidote is hydroxocobalamin in Cyanokit, turns urine red/pink since converts into Vitamin B12.

d. **Burn injury levels.**
   i. Superficial – epidermis, no blisters.
   ii. Partial-thickness – blisters, blanches.
   iii. Deep-thickness – deep dermis, cherry red, does not blanch.
   iv. Full-thickness – leathery appearance, requires grafting.
   v. Circumferential burns may require escharotomy, especially chest to allow lungs to expand.
   vi. Hand and foot – risk of contractures.

e. Zone of coagulation – most damaged, requires skin grafting. Zone of stasis – moderately damaged. Zone of hyperemia – outermost area.

f. Lund and Browder preferred, Rule of Nines, Rule of palms is 1% (includes fingers).

g. Transfer criteria – partial thickness > 10%, burns of face, hands, feet, genitalia, major joints, pre-existing medical disorders.
   i. Care during transfer - Cover with clean, dry sheet; no ice; keep patient warm, do no debride, no ointments.

h. **Burn Fluid resuscitation formulas.**
   i. Fluids prior to BSA calculation
      1. 500 ml/hour for 14 and older, 250 ml/hour for 6-13 years of age, 125 ml/hour for 5 years and younger.
   ii. Based on partial, deep, and full-thickness burns (not superficial).
   iii. LR is fluid of choice, half of total amount in first 8 hours from time of burn.
   iv. American Burn Association (ABA) guidelines, ACE it!
      1. **A**dult thermal = 2ml x kg x BSA for 24-hour calculation
      2. **C**hild thermal = 3ml x kg x BSA for 24-hour calculation (< 14 years of age)
      3. **E**lectrical = 4ml x kg x BSA for 24-hour calculation
   v. Adjust fluid based on urinary output, need 0.5-1.0 ml/kg/hour adult (30-60 cc/hour), 1-2ml/kg/hour in peds. Infuse D5LR maintenance on pediatric patients to maintain glucose levels.
   vi. Parkland formula is only **considered** for adult thermal burns= 4ml x kg x BSA for 24-hour calculation.

i. **Electrical burns**
   i. Do not document entrance and exit wound, just point of contact.
   ii. Hand-to-hand – increased risk of heart damage since across the heart, risk of V Fib or asystole.
   iii. Risk of rhabdomyolysis and acute kidney injury so increase IVFs to get UO at least 75-100 ml/hr.

j. **Lightning strike** – lace or feathering appearance (Lichtenberg figures). Cataracts develop over time.

k. **Chemical burns** – first goal is to reduce exposure to others, so don personal protective equipment first.
   i. If gasoline, decontaminate outside.
   ii. Decontaminate – Hot zone only for suited, warm for decontamination, cold for treatment.
   iii. Brush off dry chemicals (lime powder).
   iv. Hydrofluoric acid – calcium to inactivate fluoride.
   v. Asphalt (tar) – if HOT, cool immediately. apply fat emollient (petroleum ointment) only after cooling if instructed by burn center. Tar removal should occur at burn center.

l. **Radiation exposure** - S/S: nausea, vomiting, diarrhea, malaise, anorexia, GI bleed; skin red, but without blisters. Removing clothing can decrease contamination by 90%. Key is time, distancing, and shielding.

Special Considerations - 25 Questions

1. **Psychosocial**
    a. Family-centered care and presence - need a clear policy and plan in place for family presence.
    b. Family death notification – **RESPOND** mnemonic – Reassure, Establish rapport, Support, manage Pain, Offer hope, Never deliver bad news alone, Determine the family's needs.
        i. Trauma is unexpected, family cannot problem-solve, interferes with coping.
        ii. Delivering bad news - Talk to them in a private space. Assess pre-existing coping mechanisms. Ask what they already know. "We did everything we could. I am sorry, but the injuries were too severe, and he died." Expect shock and denial. "No, he is not dead." Allow them to talk, non-judgmental listening.
    c. Grief reaction – Denial first "Can't be", Anger, Bargaining, Depression, Acceptance (home from rehab, understands need for wheelchair and ramp).)
    d. Human responses to grief - somatic – physical symptoms like nausea and headache; cognitive – helplessness; affective – guilt and depression; behavioral-crying.
    e. Traumatic Stress Disorder
        i. Acute Stress Disorder (ASD) begins immediately after the traumatic event and resolves within 3 months.
        ii. The typical onset of PTSD is 3 months after event and lasting > 1 month.
        iii. S/S: vivid memories/flashbacks, sleep disorders, angry outbursts, nightmares, hyper startle response, isolation/numb, palpitations, difficulty breathing.
        iv. Place the patient in a low stimulus area. Announce yourself before entering the patient room. The patient is better if they can concentrate.
2. **Shock physiology**
    a. Hemodynamics of shock - Cardiac output = heart rate x stroke volume. Stroke volume is dependent on preload or volume – CVP (right) and PAOP (left), afterload (resistance – SVR), and contractility. CVP – 2-6, PAOP 8-12, SVR 800-1200 normal.
    b. SvO_2 and $ScvO_2$ (oxygen delivery to cells) are low in all shock states.
    c. Baroreceptors sense a decrease in stretching and stimulate the sympathetic nervous system. Chemoreceptors detect low oxygen and increase RR and BP. The sympathetic nervous system releases catecholamines from adrenal glands, increasing HR and contractility, vasoconstriction, and glycogenolysis. Hypoperfusion of the kidneys triggers renin to activate angiotensin I into angiotensin II and stimulates aldosterone and antidiuretic hormone (ADH).
    d. DX: Serum lactate, anion gap, base deficit, and pH to assess the degree of acidosis and oxygen debt.
    e. Initial blood sugar is elevated from sympathetic nervous system response - gluconeogenesis.
    f. Beta-blockers may mask the early signs of shock, such as tachycardia and diaphoresis.
    g. Pulse pressure = SBP-DBP. Pulse pressure narrows in early shock, widens in increased ICP.
    h. **Lethal triad** of trauma – hypothermia (so warm fluids), acidosis (low pH), coagulopathy (do not dilute blood with more than 1 liter of warmed isotonic crystalloids). Now includes hypocalcemia (lethal diamond).
    i. Stages of shock
        i. Compensated - restlessness, narrow pulse pressure.
        ii. Decompensated/progressive - decreased LOC, HR > 100 bpm, thready pulses, cool skin, hypotension.
        iii. Irreversible/refractory - unresponsive, bradycardia, marked hypotension.
    j. **Classes of shock**
        i. Class I – pulse < 100, pulse pressure narrowed.
        ii. Class II – pulse 100-120.
        iii. Class III – hypotension.
        iv. Class IV – pulse > 140.
    k. **Permissive hypotension** – to avoid exsanguination and dislodgement of clots, while maintaining vital organ perfusion. Mostly used in pelvic fracture and abdominal penetrating injury. No permissive hypotension in pediatrics, elderly, or traumatic brain injury.
    l. **Shock index** – HR divided by SBP (normal 0.5-0.7) – 0.9 poor prognosis.

3. **Shock types**
    a. **Hypovolemic** – (volume loss) "Empty Tank"- hemorrhagic or non-hemorrhagic (burns). Replace the type of volume lost, like blood products.
    b. **Cardiogenic** – "Pump Pooped" - heart damage from blunt cardiac injury. TX: inotropic support, controlled fluid administration, and antidysrhythmics.
    c. **Obstructive** – (mechanical obstruction) - cardiac tamponade, tension pneumothorax, abdominal compartment syndrome, supine vena cava syndrome in OB, massive PE, excessive PEEP, air embolism. TX: relieve the obstruction, position pregnant patient on side, adjust ventilator PEEP settings.
    d. **Distributive** (maldistribution of blood) "Pipe Problem", vasodilation – decreased systemic vascular resistance – SVR.
        i. **Neurogenic** – bradycardia (or lack of tachycardia) due to unopposed parasympathetic vagal activity, bradypnea, hypotension. TX: Augment vascular tone with IVF's and Norepinephrine.
        ii. **Septic** - TX: CBC, blood cultures, antibiotics, IVFs, and Norepinephrine.
        iii. **Anaphylactic** – vasodilation and bronchospasm. TX: Epinephrine 0.3-0.5 mg IM, histamine blockers, IVFs.
4. **Shock management strategies** (Damage control resuscitation)
    a. Balanced (hypotensive) resuscitation – limit crystalloids to 1 liter in adults so you do not "pop the clot".
    b. Massive transfusion protocol – Initially start large bore 16-gauge peripheral IV, then insert 8.5 Fr Cordis or Arrow central line femoral or internal jugular for rapid infuser. Use plain xylocaine to control pain in intraosseous use.
    c. **Hemostatic resuscitation** - PRBCs + Platelets + FFP at 1:1:1 ratio and control bleeding.
        i. Universal RBC donor is O negative, plasma AB negative is universal donor. Albumin does not require type/crossmatch.
            1. Can give Rh+ to males and postmenopausal women.
        ii. Each unit of PRBC's (250-300 mL) increases hemoglobin by 1 g/dl, hematocrit by 3%. (pg. 83) Each unit of platelets increases levels by 5-10,000.
        iii. Citrate in PRBCs binds with calcium rendering it inactive – need to replace calcium; pH of packed cells is 7.1 so causes acidosis, so consider whole blood.
        iv. TRALI – transfusion-related acute lung injury – acute onset of hypoxemia during transfusion or within 6 hours of transfusion.
    d. Pediatric – rapid infusion of 20 ml/kg of warmed crystalloid solution over 5-10 minutes with a three-way stopcock and a 20 ml syringe. Whole blood, packed RBC's, platelets, and plasma bolused at 10 ml/kg. No rapid infuser if weight < 40 kgs.
    e. Damage control surgery limited to under 90 minutes, not definitive repair. Definitive repair when stable and warm.
    f. Tranexamic acid (TXA) is an antifibrinolytic, so clots do not dissolve. The initial dose is 1 gram/ 100 mL NS/LR over 10 minutes, followed by 1 gram in 500 mL over 8 hours. Given IV or IO.
    g. TEG and ROTEM are point-of-care testing to evaluate the efficiency of blood clotting, platelet function, clot strength, and fibrinolysis.
    h. REBOA stops hemorrhage within the chest at zone 1, within the abdomen and pelvis at zone 3.
    i. Tourniquets and hemostatic dressings (CELOX and Quick Clot) to hasten clotting.
    j. Resuscitation Goals (to restore tissue oxygenation)
        i. Urine output of 0.5 ml/kg/hour in adults, CVP of 2-6 mmHg, PAOP of 8-12, CI of 2.5-4.0. Normal lactate and base deficit of -2 to +2.
5. **Sepsis Continuum**
    a. SIRS (2 or more of the following) – temperature > 38 or < 36, HR > 90, RR > 20, WBC > 12,000 or < 4,000 or > 10% bands. Sepsis – SIRS plus suspected or known source. Septic shock – requires vasopressors to increase BP.
6. **Multiple Organ Dysfunction** (MODS) – ARDS (patchy infiltrates), renal failure (Creatinine > 2), liver failure (bilirubin > 2), DIC (platelets < 100K, decreased fibrinogen and H&H, increased d-dimer, FSP, and PT/PTT).
    a. Prevention of MODS - insulin to keep blood sugar < 150 and start nutrition within 24 hours.
7. **Ventilator-associated pneumonia** (VAP) - elevate HOB 30 to 45 degrees and provide frequent oral care with chlorhexidine oral care to prevent VAP.

8. **Acute lung injury** (ALI) and **acute respiratory distress** (ARDS) – 24-48 hours post injury, refractory hypoxemia. Mechanically ventilate with low tidal volume of 6 ml/kg and PEEP of 10-15 mmHg, prone positioning.
9. **Deep vein thrombosis** (DVT) – ambulate early, administer low-molecular weight heparin, and apply compression stockings or use intermittent pneumatic compression devices to prevent.
10. **DIC** labs – decreased platelet count, fibrinogen, and hemoglobin/hematocrit. Elevated D-dimer and fibrin degradation products. Prolonged PT and PTT.
11. **CAUTI** – prevent by performing daily audit to remove catheters ASAP. Properly secure catheter.
12. **SBIRT** (screening, brief intervention, and referral for treatment) identifies at-risk alcohol and drug-addicted individuals who may benefit from in-depth evaluation. Alcohol and drugs are frequently contributing factors to trauma. Screen all admitted patients > 12 years of age.
13. **Forensics**
    a. Documentation – "direct quotes", facts only, do NOT document entrance and exit wound.
    b. Place evidence in paper bags, not plastic due to molding from moisture, degrading DNA.
    c. Do not cut clothes through stains. Preserve paint chips from car versus pedestrian, folded in paper.
    d. Use gloved hand or rubber-tipped forceps to retrieve bullet casing.
    e. Follow chain of custody – limit number of staff in ownership of forensic evidence. Preferred if nurse who collects evidence turns it over to the law enforcement officer, documenting their name, agency, and badge number to best ensure integrity of evidence.
14. **Autism Spectrum Disorder** – more sensitive to sound and light, so decrease stimulus, and get caregivers involved, have noise-cancelling headphones, sunglasses, and weighted blanket available.
15. **Bariatric** – ramped position for intubation due to increased risk of aspiration. Rocuronium based on ideal body weight. Succinylcholine based on total body weight.
16. **Geriatric** – reverse anticoagulants and assess shock index. Assess for maltreatment, restraint marks. Low energy falls from medications, syncope, improper footwear, low lighting, altered vision.
17. **Pediatric** – assess for maltreatment, burns with lines of demarcation (sock-like or glove-like burn). Be honest about pain.

Continuum of Care - 15 Questions

1. **Prehospital care** – scene safety is priority, so if off duty trauma nurse drives up on scene, do not get injured yourself.
    a. CDC Field Triage criteria to transfer to trauma center (listing most common scenarios on exam)
        i. Physiologic (GCS < 13, SBP <90)
        ii. Anatomic (pelvic fracture or paralysis)
        iii. Mechanism of injury (adult fall > 20 feet, child > 10 feet)
        iv. Special considerations (SBP <110 in adult > 65, anticoagulant use).
2. **MVC Sequence** – 1st is car into object, 2nd impact is occupant into car interior, 3rd impact is organs into bone causing coup/contrecoup brain injuries, aorta tear from shearing.
3. **Blast injury** – Primary injury from impact, secondary fragmentation injuries, tertiary amputations.
4. **The "E's" of injury control** – Engineering (air bags, lane assist, athletic safety gear), Education (distracted driving), Enforcement (click it or ticket), Economic incentives (insurance rebates)
5. **Injury Prevention**
    a. Primary – reduces occurrences like MVC's, falls, etc.
        i. EX: advocate for bicycle lanes and speed bumps, educate on distracted driving, safe driving education, water heaters at 120 (49 degrees), check bathwater for infant 100 (38 degrees), check back seat for baby before locking car, fall prevention programs like social worker assessing home.
    b. Secondary – decreases severity of injury but does not prevent injury.
        i. EX: provide helmets and educate correct sizing, car seats, and smoke detectors, teach Stop the Bleed program.
    c. Tertiary – reduces consequences of trauma, improves patient outcomes.
        i. EX: advocate for burn centers and trauma centers, lobby for good Samaritan law, helicopter at rural facilities, dedicated trauma team, following EBP.

6. **Tertiary trauma assessment** within 24 hours of admission, when patient is awake and can describe pain, and prior to discharge with the purpose of identifying missed injuries.
7. **Complications**
   a. Pulmonary contusion risk peaks at 72 hours, mostly from rib fractures.
   b. Most pulmonary emboli occur within first 4 days – sudden onset of severe respiratory distress and hypoxemia.
   c. Fat embolism syndrome – most 24-72 hours post injury, seen post long bone fracture. Same S/S as pulmonary embolus, plus petechial rash.
   d. Temperature spike – think sepsis first.
8. **Transfer/Transport**
   a. Expedite transfer as soon as you realize patient's needs exceed your resources.
   b. Allow the family to see the patient prior to transfer if possible.
   c. Ground transport may be able to transfer in bad weather when air cannot, larger space.
   d. Rotor-wing (helicopter) – not pressured so no air splints, faster point-to-point transfer, but cannot fly in inclement weather. Great choice for shorter transport (50 miles) in critically injured.
   e. Fixed wing (airplane) is typically pressurized but needs a landing strip. Good for longer transport and may be able to fly in inclement weather.
   f. ACS criteria for transfer (listing most common scenarios on exam)
      i. Pulmonary contusion with P:F ratio < 200 (ARDS)
      ii. Grade IV or V liver injury receiving 6 units of packed RBCs.
      iii. Spinal fracture or cord deficit
   g. Burn center transfer (listing most common scenarios on exam). Dry dressings to keep warm. Wet dressings increase bacterial growth.
      i. Burn to face, hands, feet, genitalia, perineum, and major joints.
      ii. Electrical or chemical burn
      iii. Pre-existing disorders like diabetes, cardiac, COPD
      iv. Child abuse
9. **Rehabilitation** – start after stabilization.
   a. A physiatrist is a rehabilitation specialist physician, leader of the multidisciplinary team.
      i. Occupational therapy guides activities of daily living.
      ii. Physical therapy builds strength.
      iii. Speech therapy assists with swallowing and speaking.
   b. Goals are restoration to normal, compensation (alternate strategies), and/or adaptation (adapt to disability).
   c. Family involvement is key, allowing the family in decision making of rehabilitation center.
   d. Pediatrics – get child life specialist involved early.
   e. Patient showing acceptance if accepting with wheelchair ramp being installed.
10. **Advanced directives** – ask patient their wishes if alert. The durable power of attorney goes in effect when the patient cannot make their own decisions.
11. Palliative care – mitigate pain and suffering and treat symptoms.
12. **Organ donation**
    a. Contact organ procurement as soon as death is deemed imminent, best to have them discuss with family.
    b. Organ donation after brain death – IVF's and vasopressin to keep MAP > 60 mm Hg.
    c. Corneal donation– can donate up to 24 hours post death, instill artificial tears, tape eyelids closed with paper tape, keep HOB up 20 degrees, ice packs over eyes.

Professional Issues - 15 Questions

1. The **American College of Surgeons** (ACS) does not designate trauma centers, rather verifies. State or local agencies designate trauma centers.
2. **Trauma care levels**
    a. I – regional resource with 24-hour coverage, typically an academic facility that offers comprehensive care, specialties, research, and rehabilitation.
    b. II – No research requirement, but clinically equivalent to level I center, except for complex injuries such as spine or replantation capabilities.
    c. III – 24-hour ED physician, surgeon within 30 minutes, and ICU; offers prompt assessment, resuscitation, and stabilization, needs transfer agreements with levels I and II.
    d. IV – 24-hour ED physician or midlevel, stabilize, then transfer, transfer agreements with I and II.
    e. V – Rural community ED that evaluates, stabilizes, and transports patients.
3. **Trauma teams** – high performing teams use a systematic, organized approach. The team leader maintains situational awareness and communicates clearly and empowers collective input.
4. **Trauma team communication**
    a. Brief at beginning of shift to assign roles, write on chalkboard.
    b. Huddle before the patient arrives to review assignments and complete checklist.
    c. Debrief after for feedback on how to improve.
5. **Transfer of patient** – must have an accepting facility and MD, send copies of medical records with appropriate transport personnel.
6. Trauma program manager – ACS requires the position to be a full-time position with trauma in level I and II.
7. Level I and II must have 24/7 medical social worker. Levels I, II, and III must have ICU.
8. **Performance Improvement (PIPS)** – goal is monitoring, evaluation, and improving performance, with a feedback loop to for an action plan.
    a. Primary – review by PI coordinator, trauma team rounding daily to make best plan for patient.
    b. Secondary – PI coordinator asks medical director to review.
    c. Tertiary – multi-disciplinary review; Mortality and Morbidity (M&M) meetings.
    d. Quaternary – outside agency reviews for independent analysis.
9. **Performance improvement cycle** – Plan, Do, Check, Act; close the loop.
    a. Evaluate surgeon response time, diversion, delay to operating room.
    b. Change or enforce policies, education, suspension for staff who vary from standard of care.
10. **Trauma registry**
    a. Aggregate data to compare your facility outcomes to local, state, and national standards (TQIP).
    b. Demographics, prehospital information, diagnoses, treatment, costs, outcomes.
    c. Use information for PIPS, to plan injury prevention for your community, research, supports verification.
11. **Clinical practice**/Evidence-based Practice/Research
    a. Example of clinical changes - ventilator-associated events bundle, sedation vacation, DVT prophylaxis, MTP, reversal of oral anticoagulants.
    b. Quantitative – numeric (deductive); qualitative – words (inductive - interview) research.
    c. Research reliability – consistent findings when repeated.
    d. Cohort study follows TBI patients over time, shows PTSD is high in TBI.
    e. Institutional Review Board (IRB) in quantitative research to ensure subjects of research studies are treated ethically.
12. **Disaster management phases**
    a. Mitigation – hazardous vulnerability assessment to discover risks. (pg. 348)
    b. Preparedness – mutual aid agreements, stockpile supplies, START disaster drill.
    c. Response – disaster triage like START and JumpStart (RR > 45) based on RPM 30, 2, can do– red most severe (ED Nurses Role is triage) or SALT (TNCC pg. 368). Do most good for greatest number.
    d. Recovery – replenish supplies, disposal of waste, and CISM to mitigate impact and restore adaptive functioning of caregivers.
13. **CBRNE** – Chemical, Biological, Radiation, Nuclear, Explosives – wash off chemicals and radiation with soap and water.

14. **Decontamination** – chemical or radiation exposure; patient flow opposite of wind direction.
15. **Ethical principles** – autonomy (right to make own healthcare decisions), beneficence (care to the best of your ability), non-maleficence (do no harm), veracity (honesty), justice (fair and equal treatment – what EMTALA is based on)
16. **Ethical considerations**
    a. Advance Directives – ask patient if alert, has a right to be fully informed and make own decision. (Autonomy)
    b. Organ and Tissue Donation – contact organ procurement organization (OPO) as soon as death is imminent. Best if the OPO representative discusses with family.
17. Compassion fatigue/burnout – late to work, sick days, anxiety, depression. Lose empathy.
18. Secondary traumatic stress – recurring thoughts and dreams about patients (intrusion in life), sleep disturbances.
19. Coping and building resilience – seek relationships outside work, have career goals, take care of yourself, talk about stress. Promote work-life balance.
20. Critical Incident Debriefings are structured and held within 24-72 hours. They are voluntary and supports resilience by mitigating the impact.
21. Agitated Families/De-escalation – have one point-of-contact, speak in calm voice, maintain an exit strategy, actively listen, don't say "it will be OK."
22. **HIPAA** – sharing information between healthcare providers caring for the patient or for research is OK. Not appropriate to access records of patients you are not caring for.
23. **EMTALA** – provide medical screening, choose appropriate transport to higher level of care, stabilize to the best of your ability prior to transport.
24. **Child car seat safety**
    a. Keep infant/toddler rear-facing in back seat up to age 3 if possible.
    b. Keep children ages 4-7 in front facing car seat in back seat.
    c. Keep ages 8-12 booster seat in back seat.
    d. All under age 13 in back seat per national highway traffic safety administration NHTSA guidelines.

PDB Nurse Education, LLC TCRN Resources

- American College of Surgeons. *Resources for Optimal Care of the Injured Patient. 2022.*
- Emergency Nurses Association. *Emergency Nurses Pediatric Course Provider Manual*, 6th edition, 2023
- Emergency Nurses Association. *Sheehy's Emergency Manual of Emergency Care*, 8th ed. Elsevier, 2024.
- Emergency Nurses Association. *Trauma Nursing Core Curriculum,* 9th ed., 2024.

This Study Guide is registered with the Board of Certification for Emergency Nursing (BCEN®); however, they do not endorse any resource or have a proprietary relationship with any publishing company.

A. Head & Neck Questions (33 Questions) – 43 Sample Questions

1. A 23-year-old patient involved in a roll-over motor vehicle collision (MVC) presents to the trauma bay with a Glascow Coma Score (GCS) of 8. The trauma nurse performs the trauma assessment in the correct order, so which of the following activities would be carried out after removal of the patient's clothing?
    a. Manual cervical spine stabilization
    b. Obtaining a full set of vital signs
    c. Placement of intravenous lines
    d. Assessment of pupillary response

B - Obtaining a full set of vital signs. Rapidly assess for and intervene for life-threatening injuries in the primary survey (ABCDE with resuscitation adjuncts FG) and identifies all injuries in a systematic manner in the secondary survey (H-I). J is for "just keep monitoring." The act of obtaining a full set of vital signs is under resuscitative adjuncts and would be completed after exposure. (TNCC 9th edition Chapter 4 Initial Assessment).

Trauma Initial Assessment

- **A**cross the room assessment for uncontrolled hemorrhage, **A**irway and **A**lertness with simultaneous cervical spine stabilization
- **B**reathing and Ventilation
- **C**irculation and Control of Bleeding
- **D**isability "Da Brain"
- **E**xposure and Environmental Control
- **F**ull set of vitals and **F**amily Presence
- **G**et adjuncts and **G**ive comfort
    - **L** = Labs (TXM, ABG, lactate)
    - **M** = Monitor (Cardiac)
    - **N** = Nasogastric or OG consideration
    - **O** = Oxygenation and Ventilation (oximetry) and ET CO_2 capnography
    - **P** = Pain assessment and management
- **H**istory and **H**ead-to-toe assessment
- **I**nspect posterior surfaces
- **J**ust keep reevaluating – A-I

2. A toddler who recognizes his parents, but will not respond to the nurse's requests is listed as which of the following when assessing mental status using the AVPU mnemonic?
    a. A for alert
    b. V for verbal
    c. P for painful
    d. U for unresponsive

A – A for alert. Toddlers may be cautious of strangers, and may not respond to healthcare provider commands, which is a normal response. (TNCC pgs. 43-44 and 275)

3. The nurse is performing a Glasgow Coma Score (GCS) assessment on a head trauma patient. His eyes open to cuticle pressure, his best verbal response is incomprehensible sounds, and he exhibits flexion (decorticate posturing). What is this patient's GCS?
    a. 6
    b. 7
    c. 8
    d. 9

B – 7/15. The **GCS** score ranges from 3 to 15 and provides a measure of the patient's level of consciousness as well as a predictor of morbidity and mortality after brain injury. This patient receives a 2 for best eye opening (to pressure), a 2 for best verbal response (incomprehensible words), and a 3 for best motor response (flexion), totaling **7 out of 15**. GCS is limited due to sedation, fractures, or spinal cord injury. (TNCC pgs. 121-123)

4. The emergency nurse is performing a Full Outline of Unresponsiveness (FOUR) assessment on a head trauma patient. His eyelids are closed, but open to loud voice. The patient exhibits flexion to pain. Pupil and corneal reflexes are present. The patient is not intubated and is breathing in a Cheyne-Stokes breathing pattern. What is this patient's FOUR score?
   a. 8
   b. 9
   c. 10
   d. 11

   D – 11/16. FOUR score evaluates four parameters - eye response, motor response, brainstem reflexes, and respiration. Each parameter is scored from 0-4, with 16 as best score. This patient scores 2 for eye response, 2 for motor response, 4 for brain stem reflexes, and 3 for respiration, totaling **11 out of 16**. FOUR score is more reliable than GCS in intubated patients. (TNCC pgs. 121-123)

5. A 16-year-old female is thrown from a horse and has significant facial injuries. On arrival at the emergency department (ED), she is bleeding from her nose and mouth and audible gurgling. What is the priority nursing intervention for this patient?
   a. Assisting breathing with a bag-valve-mask device
   b. Suctioning of the airway
   c. Insertion of a nasogastric (NG) tube
   d. Preparing for intubation

   B - **Suctioning of the airway takes priority over assisting breathing.** Although this patient requires a definitive airway the initial intervention is to suction and clear the airway. Do not insert a nasogastric. **"No hose in the nose,** because nobody knows where the hose goes". (TNCC pg. 44).

6. A 20-year-old patient with a self-inflicted GSW to the face presents with severe tissue loss to the mid-face and jaw. Which of the following airway management strategies is **most** appropriate?
   a. Needle cricothyrotomy
   b. Nasal intubation
   c. Surgical cricothyrotomy
   d. Bag-valve–mask ventilation

   C - Surgical cricothyrotomy is most appropriate. Patients with severe facial trauma require a surgical airway. **Surgical cricothyrotomy** allows rapid access to the trachea and oxygen/ventilation support. Perform a **needle cricothyrotomy for child < 12 years old**. Until this patient's airway is established, the patient should be positioned in a high-fowlers position. (TNCC pg. 73)

7. Your trauma center is receiving several multi-trauma patients after a building collapse. Which neuromuscular blocking agent should be avoided in patients with crush injury?
   a. Rocuronium (Zemuron)
   b. Succinylcholine (Anectine)
   c. Vecuronium (Norcuron)
   d. Pancuronium (Pavulon)

   B - Succinylcholine (Anectine) is a depolarizing agent that causes fasciculations, and is contraindicated in Guillain Barre, patients with a history of malignant hyperthermia, **crush injury**, burns > 24 hours, and **hyperkalemia**. (TNCC pg. 85)

8. A 30-year-old male is brought to the ED by the police after crashing his moped into a guardrail. After a negative head scan (CT), he is diagnosed with a concussion and admitted for observation. The nurse notices periorbital ecchymosis on exam the next morning. What is the likely source of the facial bruising?
   a. Middle fossa fracture
   b. Anterior fossa fracture
   c. Middle meningeal tear
   d. Bridging vein injury

B - Anterior fossa basilar skull fracture. S/S include cerebral spinal fluid (CSF) leakage, facial paralysis and/or hearing loss (7th and 8th nerve dysfunction). An anterior results in periorbital bruising and rhinorrhea. Middle results in mastoid ecchymosis and otorrhea. Basilar skull fractures have a high rate of infection. A middle meningeal tear is associated with an epidural hematoma. A bridging vein injury results in a subdural hematoma. (TNCC pg. 124)

9. A head trauma patient diagnosed with a basilar skull fracture has clear liquid draining from his left ear. The appropriate nursing action is to:
   a. Reposition the patient onto his right side.
   b. Test the fluid for glucose.
   c. Obtain a sample for culture.
   d. Place a gauze-wick in the patient's ear.

B - Test the fluid for glucose. Cerebral spinal fluid (CSF) contains glucose (66% of serum glucose) so check glucose if clear fluid. With a **bloody sample, a "halo test"** will dry with a dark inner ring and a lighter outer ring. Glucose testing is not reliable with a bloody sample since blood contains glucose. **Do not pack the ears or nose, allow CSF to drain through a sterile drip pad to reduce ICP**. (TNCC pgs. 124-125)

10. Which of the following statements is **INCORRECT** regarding drug-assisted intubation medications?
    a. Lidocaine may reduce the risk of rise in intracranial pressure during intubation.
    b. Etomidate is likely to cause a decrease in mean arterial pressure (MAP).
    c. Ketamine provides analgesia.
    d. Use Propofol cautiously in patients with egg/soy allergies.

B - Etomidate is not likely to cause a decrease in MAP like Midazolam and Propofol, so it is a good choice for induction in unstable trauma patients. (TNCC pg. 85)

11. A 65-year-old female fell down several stairs two weeks ago. She was examined after the fall and discharged with a diagnosis of concussion but returns today with new-onset confusion. She has a history of alcohol abuse, but confusion is a new finding. Which of the following diagnostic tests would most likely explain the cause of this patient's confusion?
    a. Electroencephalography (EEG)
    b. Brain MRI
    c. Blood ethanol level
    d. Head computed tomography (CT)

D - Head CT scan would allow rapid visualization inside the skull of any intracerebral bleeding. **Subdural hematomas (SDH) arise from tearing of the venous bridging veins** and may evolve weeks after an initial traumatic insult. Subdural hematomas appear as a "crescent-shape" on CT. Those taking **anticoagulants, chronic alcohol users, and the elderly** are at highest risk for SDH. EEG shows electrical brain activity and is used to evaluate seizure and brain death. ETOH level is helpful in those patients for whom the diagnostic cause of a decreased level of consciousness is unclear. (TNCC pgs. 127-129)

12. A 70-year-old female with a history of atrial fibrillation is diagnosed with an acute subdural hematoma after a fall. She takes Eliquis (Apixaban) daily, so the nurse prepares to administer which medication while awaiting transfer to the OR?
    a. Kcentra (Prothrombin concentrate)
    b. Protamine sulfate
    c. Andexxa (Coag factor Xa)
    d. Tranexamic acid (TXA)

C - Andexxa is the reversal agent used for Eliquis (Apixaban) and Xarelto (Rivaroxaban). Kcentra is the reversal for warfarin (coumadin). Protamine sulfate is the reversal agent for heparin. (TNCC pg. 134)

13. A 20-year-old female is transported to the ED after falling while snow-skiing, hitting the right side of her head. She was unresponsive initially, had a short period of lucidity, then became unresponsive. Her right pupil is dilated, and her pulse pressure is widening. The trauma nurse anticipates:
    a. Lumbar puncture to drain cerebral spinal fluid.
    b. Emergent burr hole and clot evacuation
    c. Ventriculostomy
    d. Endovascular coiling

B – Emergent burr holes and clot evacuation is required in epidural hematoma with uncal transtentorial herniation. Epidural hematomas are frequently from a tear of the **middle meningeal artery**. (TNCC pg. 127)

14. What is the most common initial clinical indication that intracranial pressure (ICP) is increasing?
    a. Hypotension
    b. Deteriorating level of consciousness
    c. Tachypnea
    d. Tachycardia

B - Deteriorating level of consciousness is the first clinical indication of increased ICP. If the patient is unresponsive, monitor for **widening pulse pressure** and posturing. (Sheehy 8th edition pg. 191)

15. An early sign of an uncal herniation would be?
    a. Doll's eyes reflex
    b. Ataxic breathing
    c. Paralysis below the diaphragm
    d. Ipsilateral pupil dilation

D - Ipsilateral pupil dilation. Uncal herniation is seen when the Uncas of the temporal lobe is **displaced unilaterally** over the tentorium into the posterior fossa. This causes what is called a **midline shift**. Central herniation is seen when the cerebral hemispheres are pushed downward constricting the brainstem. Herniation is associated with drastic changes in neurologic status including loss of pupillary reactivity and abnormal posturing. (TNCC pg. 129)

16. Which of the following statements is appropriate to include in the discharge information for a child who sustained a concussion while playing soccer?
    a. "Your son will need to be medically cleared before he returns to play."
    b. "Make sure you keep him up tonight to ensure he doesn't fall asleep."
    c. "Medications with caffeine can help his headaches."
    d. "Make an appointment with his pediatrician if he feels dizzy or throws up."

A - "Your son will need to be medically cleared before he returns to play." Concussion **discharge education**: Monitor the child for mentation changes. Do NOT administer narcotics, aspirin, or NSAIDs. Allow **cognitive brain rest**, do not awaken patient. If the patient develops mentation changes, pupil changes, vomiting, and/or seizures seek immediate ED intervention. **Medical clearance** should be performed by a concussion specialist prior to reentry to sport and a **graduated return to play** plan followed. (TNCC pg. 130)

17. Which of the following ranges are normal for cerebral perfusion pressure (CPP)?
    a. 0-20 mm Hg
    b. 50-70 mm Hg
    c. 60-80 mm Hg
    d. 100-120 mm Hg

C - Normal CPP = 60-80 mm Hg, some manuals list 60-100. CPP = MAP – ICP. **Keep > 60 mm Hg with increased ICP.** Hypotension, hypoxemia, and hypercarbia are associated with an increased mortality in TBI. Normal mean arterial pressure (MAP) = 90 {(DBPx2) +SBP} divided by 3. **ICP normal range is 3-15** for an adult. **Treat if ICP is sustained > 20-22 (ranges vary per text)**. (TNCC pg. 116)

18. An unhelmeted motorcyclist is admitted to trauma ICU with head injury. The left pupil is dilated and unreactive, the right pupil is 5 mm and sluggishly reactive. The GCS is 9 and ICP is 25 mm Hg. The trauma nurse knows that additional **late signs** of increased ICP may include:
    a. Narrowed pulse pressure, irregular respirations, and bradycardia.
    b. Widening pulse pressure, Cheyne-Stokes respirations, and bradycardia.
    c. Narrowed pulse pressure, Kussmaul's respirations, and tachycardia.
    d. Widening pulse pressure, tachypnea, and tachycardia.

B - Cushing's Triad = widened pulse pressure, abnormal respirations or decreased respiratory effort, and profound bradycardia. Early signs of increasing ICP include the patient requiring more stimulation for response, pupils sluggish to light, tachycardia, and hypertension. **Late signs are the patient** responding to pain only or unresponsive, fixed, or dilated pupils, posturing or no motor response, and **Cushing's Triad.** (TNCC pg. 117)

19. A patient was beaten with a baseball bat and intubated on arrival to the trauma bay due to head trauma. His initial ICP was 20, but over the last hour, his ICP has climbed to 40. He currently has an O_2 sat of 97%, CO_2 of 40, and MAP of 92 mm Hg. What emergent intervention does the trauma nurse anticipate?
    a. Administration of Norepinephrine (Levophed) to increase CPP.
    b. Administration of Mannitol (Osmitrol) IV.
    c. Administration of Labetalol to manage blood pressure.
    d. Sustained hyperventilation to facilitate CO_2 exhalation.

B - Administration of Mannitol IV. Mannitol and hypertonic saline are used to treat increased ICP. A bolus of mannitol 1 gm/kg should be given over 5 minutes. Since Mannitol is an **osmotic diuretic,** electrolytes and **serum osmolality should be monitored closely**. Mannitol may cause hypotension so it should not be given to patients with existing hypotension. **The treatment is effective if the GCS increases. Systolic BP should be maintained > 100-110 mm Hg**. (TNCC pgs. 133-135)

20. A 42-year-old female presents to the trauma bay after a fall from 30 feet with massive facial trauma with obvious fractures to both upper extremities. Head CT shows a subdural hematoma with a midline shift of 3mm. Her GCS is 3 and she remains hypotensive despite blood transfusions. The trauma nurse anticipates an order for which medication?
    a. Mannitol
    b. Hypertonic saline
    c. Solu-cortef
    d. Normal saline

B - Hypertonic saline (3%, 7.5%, 10%). Both mannitol and hypertonic saline lower increased ICP normally, but **Mannitol will not lower ICP in hypovolemia.** Since mannitol is an osmotic diuretic, it is contraindicated in patients with existing hypotension. Steroids (solu-cortef) are not indicated in head injury. (TNCC pgs. 133-135)

21. A ventilator-dependent patient with a severe traumatic brain injury (TBI) exhibits decerebrate posturing, no cough or gag reflex, hypertension, and hyperthermia. The initial CT showed no acute bleed or focal injury. A likely cause of this patient's symptoms is:
    a. Epidural hematoma (EDH)
    b. Subdural hematoma (SDH)
    c. Diffuse axonal injury (DAI)
    d. Basilar skull fracture (BSF)

C - Diffuse axonal injury (DAI) is microscopic damage to axons, diffuse white matter degeneration, global neuro dysfunction, and diffuse cerebral swelling. **DAI is caused by acceleration-deceleration of the brain** which shears the axons, causing a disconnection of cortex and brain stem. The patient will have severe neurologic deficits, but no focal lesions on cat scan (CT). An **MRI** will show diffuse microscopic hemorrhages. (TNCC pg. 130)

22. Your patient is diagnosed with diffuse axonal injury. Which intervention is appropriate to decrease intracranial pressure?
    a. Keep the patient's head in a neutral midline position.
    b. Apply a rigid cervical collar to keep the head midline.
    c. Turn the patient onto their left side to promote circulation.
    d. Elevate the head of the bed with their knees flexed.

A – **Nursing interventions to decrease intracranial pressure** include keeping the head in a neutral position, elevating the **head of the bed 30 to 45 degrees** without flexing knees, and **removing rigid cervical collars**. Speak softly and limit visitors appropriately. (TNCC pgs. 133-135)

23. Which of the following patients would **NOT** require cervical spine imaging per the Canadian C-Spine Rule?
    a. A 67-year-old involved in a low-speed rear-impact MVC at a stop sign who denies neck pain.
    b. An ambulatory 17-year-old who has tingling in his extremities after diving into a pool.
    c. A 50-year-old who was ambulatory at the scene and can actively rotate his neck 45 degrees left and right.
    d. A 20-year-old from a rear-end MVC hit by a large truck.

C – If alert and stable, **a patient who is ambulatory at any time is low risk** for cervical spine injury. If the patient can actively rotate neck 45 left and right, no cervical spine imaging or immobilization is needed. "Sixty-five, fast drive, sense deprive, image, if alive." "Sitting down and walking around, spine is fine." (TNCC pg. 224)

24. A patient from a single-car collision is transported to the ED via EMS accompanied by a law enforcement. The patient is in full spinal immobilization with a rigid cervical collar, has O_2 via NRB at 15 L, and a 20-gauge IV in the left hand with NS at 75 cc/hr. EMS reports the patient ran off the road and hit a tree with minor damage to the vehicle. Law enforcement reports a roadside breathalyzer of 0.10. Assessment reveals multiple abrasions and lacerations to the face and arms. According to NEXUS Criteria for Cervical Spine Clearance, when should the patient be removed from spinal immobilization?
    a. Following the primary and secondary assessment when no focal neurologic deficit is discovered.
    b. After the patient's blood alcohol level decreases to less than 0.08.
    c. After normal examination and negative AP and lateral radiographs.
    d. Immediately upon arrival to the ED due to the adverse effects of spinal immobilization.

C - **After normal examination and negative AP and lateral radiographs.** NEXUS Criteria includes focal **n**eurologic deficit, posterior midline cervical **s**pine tenderness, **a**lertness, **i**ntoxication, and a painful **d**istracting injury (NSAID mnemonic). (TNCC pg. 225)

25. A patient is brought to the trauma bay with a stab wound to Zone 2 of his neck. He speaks clearly and handles his secretions well. VS: HR=74, RR=16; BP=127/78, O_2 sat 97%. While awaiting transport to the OR for repair, the trauma nurse monitors the patient closely for what sign of airway compromise requiring immediate treatment?
    a. Bleeding around the injury site
    b. Ecchymosis at the injury site
    c. Rapidly increasing hematoma in the neck
    d. Abrasions to the anterior neck

C - **Rapidly increasing hematoma in the neck.** Hematomas, bruits, airway stridor, dysphonia, dysphagia, and neurologic deficits may indicate the need for emergent airway management and angiography and/or surgical intervention. **Most injuries occur in zone 2** of the neck; left sided injuries are more common because most assailants are right-handed. **Zone 1 injuries are the most lethal**. (TNCC pgs. 143-144)

26. A dirt bike rider strikes a suspended cable sustaining blunt neck trauma "clothesline injury". Which assessment finding indicates the need for emergent intervention?
    a. Ecchymosis at the injured area
    b. Anterior neck abrasions
    c. Dysphonia
    d. Coughing

C - Dysphonia (hoarseness) and dysphagia may indicate a fracture of the larynx. Blunt neck trauma patients often present stable, but the injury can quickly become emergent since there are many important anatomic structures in the neck. The neck contains airways, blood vessels, **brachial plexus**, esophagus, endocrine glands, and the spinal column. In tracheobronchial injury, airway obstruction requires emergent management with fiberoptic bronchoscopy since positive pressure ventilation may worsen the distress. You may also palpate subcutaneous emphysema and hear **"Hamman's crunch"** synchronized with the heartbeat. (TNCC pgs. 143-144)

27. You receive a patient after a fall from a deer stand. VS: HR=58, RR=24, BP=76/30 mm Hg. EMS reports a brief loss of consciousness at the scene, but the GCS is now 13. His skin is pink, warm, and dry. The nurse suspects he/she is observing?
    a. A patient in neurogenic shock, with blocked sympathetic outflow tracts.
    b. The normal vital signs of a physically fit patient.
    c. An intoxicated patient who is dehydrated after a day of drinking beer.
    d. A patient demonstrating the symptoms of Cushing's response.

A - Neurogenic shock is a form of distributive shock. S/S of neurogenic shock are **warm, dry, flushed skin** below the level of injury and cool and clammy skin above the level of injury, **bradycardia (or lack of tachycardia), hypotension**, increased RR, paraplegia, and/or quadriplegia. Treatment of neurogenic shock may include assisting breathing and **augmenting vascular tone** with intravenous fluids, **Norepinephrine, and Dopamine (positive inotrope)**. (TNCC pg. 199)

28. Which of the following functions/sensations is typically preserved in a patient with an anterior cord syndrome?
    a. Motor function
    b. Pain sensation
    c. Proprioception
    d. Temperature sensation

C - Proprioception. Anterior cord syndrome is characterized by immediate onset of **complete motor paralysis** and loss of pain and temperature sensation. The posterior column is preserved, sparing vibration sense, position sense (proprioception), deep pressure, and light touch. Anterior cord syndrome mimics complete cord syndrome and has **the worst prognosis of the incomplete injuries**, with only **10-20% recovery of motor function**. (TNCC pgs. 201-202)

29. An elderly patient is admitted after falling down a flight of stairs. He complains of weakness and tingling in his arms and can move his legs. Which cord syndrome are these findings likely related to:
    a. Anterior cord syndrome
    b. Brown-Sequard syndrome
    c. Central cord syndrome
    d. Posterior cord syndrome

C - Central cord syndrome is the most common incomplete cord injury. In elderly patients with degenerative arthritis a forced hyperextension may result in a central cord syndrome. Patients often present with **increased motor deficit in upper extremities compared to the lower extremities**, and **dysesthesia** (burning, tingling in arms and hands). It has a good prognosis, although **full functional recovery is rare** (permanent clumsy hands). (TNCC pgs. 201-202)

30. A 20-year-old male is stabbed in the back during an altercation. In Brown-Sequard syndrome, there is ipsilateral loss of what function?
    a. Pain
    b. Temperature
    c. Motor function
    d. Proprioception

C - Motor function. Brown-Sequard Syndrome (2 words – 2 sides) is a transverse hemi transection most often from **penetrating injury** (stab or gunshot wound) which results in **loss of motor function on the same side (ipsilateral) as the injury**, and loss of pain and temperature on opposite side of injury (contralateral). This syndrome has an excellent prognosis. (TNCC pgs. 202-203)

Incomplete SCI

- **A**nterior Cord
  - Loss of motor function, pain, crude touch, & temperature; retains proprioception.
- **B**rown-Sequard Syndrome *(2 words – 2 sides)*
  - Transverse hemisection (*Stab or GSW*)
  - Loss of motor function on side of injury (ipsilateral)
  - Loss of pain & temperature on opposite side of injury (contralateral)
- **C**entral Cord
  - Loss of motor & sensory function, more pronounced in arms than legs *(walk to table, but can't eat)*
- Posterior Cord
  - Loss of proprioception, vibration, fine touch, & fine pressure. Intact motor function

31. Excluding brain herniation, why is hyperventilation to achieve a $PaCO_2 < 35$ mm Hg contraindicated in patients with trauma brain injury?
    a. It increases seizure risk, causing secondary brain injury.
    b. It increases cerebral metabolic demand.
    c. It decreases venous return to the brain.
    d. It causes cerebral vasoconstriction which decreases cerebral blood flow.

D – Hyperventilation causes cerebral vasoconstriction which decreases cerebral flow, so maintain CO_2 between 35-40 mm Hg. Fever increases metabolic demand. (TNCC pg. 118)

32. Which of the following assessment findings is seen in spinal shock?
    a. Bradycardia
    b. Flash capillary refill
    c. Flaccidity
    d. Brudzinski's sign

C – Transient loss of muscle tone (flaccidity) with loss of reflexes at or below the level of the injury is seen in spinal shock. Bradycardia is seen in neurogenic shock. Flash capillary refill is seen in hyperdynamic septic shock. Brudzinski's sign is seen in meningitis. (TNCC pg. 199)

33. To assess for spinal injury, ask the patient to wiggle their fingers and toes, and lift their arms and legs. Extending and flexing arms requires innervation up to what level?
    a. C5 to C7
    b. L2 to L4
    c. L4 to L5
    d. S3 to S5

A – C5 to C7 innervation is required to extend and flex arms. C3,4,5 keep your diaphragm alive. C5,6,7, raise your arms to heaven. L2 to L4 is required to extend and flex legs. L4 to L5 is required to flex foot and extend toes. S3 to S5 is required to tighten the anus. (TNCC pg. 190)

34. A patient involved in a bar fight is diagnosed with an orbital fracture. Clinical findings are likely to include:
    a. Blood in the anterior chamber of the eye and increased intraocular pressure (IOP)
    b. Limited upward gaze and diplopia
    c. Painless loss of a visual field and perception of floaters
    d. Severe eye pain and a cloudy cornea

B - Limited upward gaze (entraps cranial nerve III oculomotor), **diplopia** (double vision), and infraorbital hypesthesia are seen in orbital fracture. **Avoid Valsalva maneuver, straining, or blowing nose**. (TNCC pgs. 132-134)

35. A 19-year-old male playing paintball without eye protection c/o a reddish hue to his vision and is diagnosed with a 20% hyphema by ophthalmology. Which of the following statements by the patient indicates successful discharge teaching?
    a. "I'll return to the ED immediately if the pain gets worse."
    b. "I will lie supine to sleep."
    c. "I will take ibuprofen if the pain is severe since I am a recovering from opioid addiction."
    d. "I'll follow up with the eye doctor in 5 days."

A - Return to the ED immediately if pain gets worse. A hyphema is a collection of **blood in the anterior chamber** due to severe intraocular trauma. Hyphemas can re-bleed leading to loss of vision. Rebleeding usually occurs in the first 5 days (3-5 days highest risk) after injury. D/C education: Instruct the patient to sleep with the head elevated approximately **30°** to decrease intraocular pressure but do not lean forward. **NSAIDS and aspirin are contraindicated** as they increase bleeding. They should be reevaluated by an ophthalmologist daily. (Sheehy 8th edition pgs. 231-232)

36. A teardrop-shaped pupil with leakage of vitreous humor is most associated with which eye injury?
    a. Orbital fracture
    b. Globe rupture
    c. Hyphema
    d. Retrobulbar hematoma

B - Globe rupture is characterized by an irregular pupil, periorbital ecchymosis, decreased visual acuity and extraocular movements, deep eye pain, and nausea. (TNCC pgs. 132-134)

37. A patient with a stick impaled in his eye has vitreous hemorrhage. The following are appropriate treatments, **EXCEPT**:
    a. Secure the stick in place and shield the eye.
    b. Patch the unaffected eye to minimize consensual movement.
    c. Instill tetracaine eye drops.
    d. Update tetanus immunization.

C – Treatment of globe rupture includes securing impaled objects, shielding the affected eye, patching the unaffected eye to minimize consensual movement, keeping the patient NPO, updating tetanus immunization, and preparing the patient for surgery. **Stabilize, do not remove impaled objects, and do not administer eye drops**. (TNCC pgs. 132-134)

38. Which facial fracture results in trismus, epistaxis, and loss of malar eminence?
    a. Maxillary fracture
    b. Mandibular fracture
    c. Orbital blowout fracture
    d. Zygoma fracture

D – In **zygoma fracture** there is deformity to the infraorbital rim with flattening of the cheek (loss of malar eminence), swelling, ecchymosis, trismus, and diplopia. Patients should be instructed to avoid blowing their nose. (Sheehy 8th edition pg. 225)

39. What is the treatment for a retrobulbar hematoma?
    a. Ice packs to the orbit for 48 hours.
    b. Topical anesthetic
    c. Lateral canthotomy
    d. Oral antibiotics

C – Emergency decompression via lateral canthotomy is the treatment for a retrobulbar hematoma. Intraocular pressures are frequently > 40 mm Hg (normal intraocular pressure < 20 mm Hg). Mannitol may be administered. (TNCC pgs. 132-134)

40. Children under age two who meet the PECARN criteria for head CT include:
    a. Child acting normally per parent.
    b. No loss of consciousness.
    c. Palpable skull fracture.
    d. No history of vomiting.

C - Palpable skull fracture, altered mental status, worsening symptoms, vomiting, and headache are components of PECARN (Pediatric Emergency Care Applied Research Network). (TNCC pg. 284)

41. A 16-year-old patient presents after a cleaning solution is splashed in his left eye. The priority nursing intervention is:
    a. Measurement of bilateral ocular pH.
    b. Copious irrigation with NS or LR.
    c. Snellen chart visual acuity assessment.
    d. Contacting his parents for permission to treat.

B - Copious irrigation with NS or LR (lactated ringers). Ocular burn severity correlates to exposure duration and the causative agent, and immediate **initiation of copious irrigation has the greatest impact on prognosis**. Acids= bleach, vinegar. **Alkalis** = cement, anhydrous ammonia, lime, tar, drain cleaner. Use NS or LR at body temperature (37 C). Irrigate until measurement of the eye pH stays at neutral level (**7.0-7.4**) for 30 minutes. (TNCC pgs. 132-134)

42. A patient has a pyramidal maxillary bone fracture involving the mid-face. Assessment findings include massive facial edema, nasal fracture, and malocclusion. This fracture is known as a:
    a. Le Fort I
    b. Le Fort II
    c. Le Fort III
    d. Zygomatic fracture

B - Le Fort II is **pyramidal shaped fracture** with transverse detachment of maxilla, fracture at bridge of **nose**, fracture through lacrimal and ethmoid bones; epistaxis, malocclusion, and lengthening of face. **Le Fort I is a** transverse detachment of the entire **maxilla above the teeth**, malocclusion, **lip laceration**. **Le Fort III is a** free-floating segment of mid-face; **craniofacial disjunction** - involves maxilla, zygomatic arch, orbits, and cranial base bones; malocclusion, immense swelling. (TNCC pgs. 131-132)

43. In which of the following facial fractures is airway assessment **most** vital because the tongue can lose control and occlude the airway?
    a. Mandibular fracture
    b. Orbital cavity fracture
    c. LeFort III
    d. Zygomatic fracture

A - Mandibular fracture is characterized by malocclusion, trismus, drooling, and paresthesia of the lower jaw. Keep the patient in **high fowlers position**, suctioning to keep airway clear, and prepare to secure airway. (TNCC pg. 132)

B. **Trunk Trauma Questions (37 Questions) – 48 Sample Questions**

1. An unrestrained driver involved in a frontal-impact MVC presents with dyspnea, hemoptysis, Hamman's crunch, and subcutaneous emphysema. Which of the following is the most likely explanation for these finding?
    a. Alveolar rupture
    b. Bleb rupture
    c. Tracheobronchial rupture
    d. Diaphragm rupture

   C - Tracheobronchial rupture may occur when blunt thoracic trauma increases pressure against a closed glottis. Airway management should be performed via **fiberoptic bronchoscopy** to prevent additional tearing or emergency cricothyrotomy. One-lung ventilation may be required. (TNCC pgs. 146 & 151)

2. A 39-year-old male arrives in the trauma bay after being stabbed in the chest. VS: HR=144, RR=26, BP=88/58. What is the critical diagnostic test for this patient?
    a. Diagnostic peritoneal lavage (DPL)
    b. Portable chest x-ray
    c. Focused Assessment Sonography for Trauma (FAST)
    d. CT scan of the chest and neck

   C - FAST. If assessment findings lead to a suspicion of uncontrolled internal bleeding (tachycardic, hypotensive) get a FAST exam to detect the presence of pericardial blood (cardiac tamponade) and heart wall motion. This patient is unstable (tachycardic, hypotensive) so he is not a candidate for CT. DPL is used to assess blood in the peritoneal cavity. **FAST exam is used to examine the pericardial sac, hepatorenal fossa, splenorenal fossa, and pelvis**. (TNCC pg. 149)

3. A farmer is kicked in the chest by a cow and presents with severe respiratory distress. VS: HR=156, RR=46, O_2 sat 78%, and BP 80/40 and worsens with inspiration. Breath sounds are absent on the right with tracheal deviation to the left. The **priority** intervention is:
    a. Endotracheal intubation
    b. Infusion of packed red blood cells.
    c. Chest radiographs
    d. Emergent needle decompression

   D - Emergent needle decompression. Tension pneumothorax requires emergent needle decompression "**needle-thoracostomy**." Location for decompression is commonly 2nd intercostal space (ICS) mid-clavicular line or 5th ICS mid-axillary line. **Improvement indicated by normalization of vital signs**. (TNCC pg. 147)

4. A farmer kicked by a bull has chest pain unrelieved by nitrates. He is tachycardic with ST segment elevation in V1-V3, and hypotensive. Troponin and CK are elevated. The nurse suspects:
    a. Blunt cardiac injury
    b. Posterior MI
    c. Tension pneumothorax
    d. Anterior wall ischemia

   A - Blunt cardiac injury causes chest pain, **sinus tachycardia, PVC's, ST segment elevation, and elevation of CK and troponin.** The right ventricle is the most common heart chamber injured. ST segment elevation in V1-V3 may be indicative of anterior injury not ischemia. Cardiac ischemia would show ST depression and negative isoenzymes. Posterior MI reveals ST segment depression in V1 & V2. The care for blunt cardiac injury is supportive, including **cardiac monitoring** for at least 24 hours, serial troponins, pain control. (TNCC pg. 157)

5. An older adult fell on the sidewalk, incurring fractures of the right 5th & 6th ribs. Which of the following is the priority intervention during this patient's hospitalization?
   a. Rib plating and repair to secure ribs.
   b. Massive transfusion protocol to replace lost blood.
   c. Adequate analgesia to promote adequate chest expansion and depth of respiration.
   d. Chest tube insertion at the right 5th ICS, MCL.

   C - Adequate analgesia to promote adequate chest expansion and depth of respiration. Complications of rib fractures, particularly in older adults and those with COPD, can be deadly. The treatment for rib fractures includes **pain management** with nerve blocks, xylocaine patches, and medications; incentive spirometry; and early ambulation (TNCC pg. 152)

6. A helmeted 35-year-old male was ejected from his motorcycle, striking a tree. He is complaining of right-sided chest pain and shortness of breath. Your exam reveals decreased breath sounds and paradoxical chest movement on the right side. VS: HR=142, RR=38, BP=82/60, O_2 sat 90% on a NRB at 15 L/minute. What is the **priority** management of this patient?
   a. Emergent surgical fixation of the ribs.
   b. Ensure adequate oxygenation and ventilation.
   c. Infuse 3 liters of NS immediately to increase BP.
   d. Chest tube placement at the 5th ICS on the right side.

   B - Ensure adequate oxygenation and ventilation. A **flail chest** occurs when two or more adjacent ribs are fractured in two or more places resulting in a free-floating segment of ribs. As the patient breathes in, the flail segment is sucked inward, and on exhalation the segment will push outward, known as **paradoxical chest movement** or **"see-saw" respirations**. S/S: respiratory distress, and pneumothorax and/or hemothorax as the rib fracture edges injure adjacent tissues, vessels, and nerves. TX: includes **adequate ventilation**, possible intubation to avoid hypoxia, and pain control. **Pulmonary contusion** is a common concurrent injury. While ensuring adequate ventilation, prepare the patient for surgical rib fixation. (TNCC pgs. 152-153)

7. A patient with blunt chest trauma is intubated due to respiratory distress. His respiratory rate and peak inspiratory pressures (PIP) are increasing, while his O_2 sat is decreasing. Crackles are auscultated throughout both lung fields. Which diagnosis is most reflective of this patient's presentation?
   a. Hemothorax
   b. Myocardial contusion
   c. Pulmonary contusion
   d. Diaphragmatic injury

   C - Pulmonary contusion starts in 24-48 hours and **peaks at 72 hours post insult**, resulting in respiratory distress and hypoxemia, which may progress to refractory hypoxemia (ARDS). The treatment for ARDS (acute respiratory distress syndrome) is **alveolar recruitment** by adding PEEP 10 to 15 mmHg. (TNCC pgs. 156-157)

8. Which of the following hemodynamic support strategies is most appropriate in the care of a stable patient diagnosed with pulmonary contusion?
   a. Rapid infusion of crystalloid solution.
   b. Judicious use of IV fluids.
   c. Transfusion with packed RBCs.
   d. Administration of FFP.

   B - Judicious use of IV fluids. Capillary blood leaks into lungs leading to pulmonary edema. Excess fluid administration increases the risk of the patient going into **ARDS**. Maintain SpO_2 94-98% and prepare for intubation and mechanical ventilation with low tidal volume and PEEP of 10 to 15 mmHg. (TNCC pg. 157)

9. Which of the following findings would be consistent with the diagnosis of hemothorax?
    a. Dullness to percussion, absent breath sounds on the affected side.
    b. Hyperresonance to percussion, absent breath sounds on affected side.
    c. Paradoxical chest wall movement, SQ emphysema.
    d. Dysphagia, bowel sounds audible in thoracic cavity.

A - Dullness to percussion, with absent breath sounds on affected side. Hyperresonance is heard in air filled space (pneumothorax), dullness from fluid (hemothorax). Paradoxical chest wall movement is seen in flail chest, bowel sounds in chest in ruptured diaphragm. **Immediate blood return of 1000-1500 ml or 200 ml/hour for 3-4 hours is an indication for surgical intervention, so report to the trauma surgeon.** (TNCC pg. 156)

10. An unstable patient with blunt trauma to the right upper chest is brought to a community ED. The patient is intubated, 2 large bore IVs are started, and a chest tube is inserted at the 5th ICS. VS: HR=138 bpm, RR=36, BP=76/50. 1600 mL of blood has drained out of the chest tube in the first 20 minutes. Which of the following interventions is indicated while awaiting critical care transfer to the trauma center?
    a. Needle thoracotomy to allow for chest expansion.
    b. Consider autotransfusion of shed chest blood.
    c. Insertion of a second chest tube to assist in evacuation of the massive hemothorax.
    d. Pericardiocentesis to evaluate for cardiac tamponade.

B - Consider autotransfusion of shed chest blood. The primary interventions for a massive hemothorax (> 1500 mL of blood) are balanced resuscitation and chest tube insertion. **Advantages of autotransfusion** include quick availability (no cross-typing), warm blood, no disease transmission, increased oxygen carrying capacity, and decreased risk of contamination. Autotransfusion is mostly used for blunt trauma due to the risk of infection in penetrating injury. For patients who continue to bleed after an **initial blood loss of > 1000-1500 mL or with blood loss of 200 mL/hour for 2-4 hours a thoracotomy** may be indicated. (TNCC pg. 156)

11. A confused patient pulls out his chest tube. What is the nurse's immediate action?
    a. Quickly replace the chest tube in the same position.
    b. Cover the wound with an occlusive dressing taped on 3 sides.
    c. Cover the wound with an occlusive dressing taped on 4 sides.
    d. Cover the wound with a non-occlusive dressing.

B - Cover the wound (temporarily) with an occlusive (non-porous) dressing applied at end-exhalation and taped on 3 sides. An open chest wound from a removed chest tube is the same as an open pneumothorax **(air leak syndrome)**. Monitor the patient closely since air may be sucked in, but NOT released, resulting in a tension pneumothorax. If this occurs, remove the dressing immediately. (TNCC pg. 154)

12. A water-seal chest drainage system is noted to have continuous bubbling in the water chamber. This could be a sign of a/an:
    a. Tension pneumothorax
    b. Hematoma development
    c. Air leak
    d. Lung re-expansion

C - Intermittent bubbling in the water chamber is a normal finding, but **continuous bubbling is an indicator of an air leak**. Assess chest drainage systems by using the **FOCA** mnemonic – Fluctuation, Output, Color of drainage, Air leak present. (TNCC pgs. 159-160)

13. Tidaling in the water-seal chamber is a:
    a. Normal finding
    b. Sign of an air leak
    c. Indicator of a displaced chest tube
    d. Sign of a pneumothorax

A - **Tidaling in the water-seal chamber can be a normal finding** and may be seen when the patient exhales, laughs, or coughs. Assess chest drainage systems by using the **FOCA** mnemonic – **F**luctuation, **O**utput, **C**olor of drainage, **A**ir leak present. (TNCC pgs. 159-160)

14. Clamping of the chest tube during transport is contraindicated since it may cause:
    a. Blood clots
    b. Tension pneumothorax
    c. ARDS development
    d. Air leak

B – **Tension pneumothorax.** Clamping the chest tube for transport or any other extended periods of time is contraindicated due to the increased intrathoracic pressure that can lead to tension pneumothorax development. (TNCC pg. 160)

15. The sudden loss of the $ETCO_2$ capnography waveform is an indicator of:
    a. Return of spontaneous circulation (ROSC)
    b. Disconnected or occluded endotracheal (ET) tube.
    c. Bronchospasm
    d. Muscle relaxants wearing off.

B - A sudden loss of waveform is an indication of a disconnected circuit or an occluded ET tube. ROSC suddenly increases $ETCO_2$ during CPR. Bronchospasm results in a "shark-fin" appearance. Muscle relaxants wearing off results in a cleft in the waveform. (TNCC pgs. 80-83)

16. A patient with severe pulmonary contusions after an MVC is intubated and mechanically ventilated. Immediate capnography shows a CO_2 of 38 mmHg. Two hours later, the CO_2 reading is 54mmHg. The trauma nurse's knowledge of physiology confirms he/she should:
    a. Increase the patient's ventilation rate.
    b. Decrease the patient's ventilation rate.
    c. Increase the positive end expiratory pressure (PEEP).
    d. Decrease the positive end expiratory pressure (PEEP).

A - Increase the patient's ventilation rate. The normal range for CO_2 is 35-45 mmHg. The patient with a CO_2 of 54 mmHg is retaining excessive CO_2 and increasing the rate will help blow off the excess CO_2. The use of waveform capnography is an inexpensive, noninvasive, rapid, and reliable method to detect abnormalities in the critically ill patient, i.e. (**DOPE mnemonic** – **D**isplacement of ET tube, **O**bstruction of tube, **P**neumothorax, **E**quipment failure. (TNCC pg. 77)

17. A patient with right fourth and fifth rib fractures should be monitored closely for signs/symptoms of:
    a. Great vessel injury
    b. Brachial plexus injury
    c. Liver injury
    d. Pulmonary contusion

D – Ribs 4 to 9 are the most common ribs fractured and associated with underlying **pulmonary contusion** and blunt cardiac injury. Fractures of ribs 1 and 2 are associated with great vessel and brachial plexus injuries. Lower rib fractures 9 to 12 are associated with liver, spleen, and renal injury. (TNCC pgs. 156-157)

18. Diagnostic tests on a patient from a rollover motor vehicle collision (MVC) reveal fractures of the left 1st and 2nd ribs. The most critical concurrent injury is:
    a. Liver injury
    b. Great vessel injury
    c. Spleen injury
    d. Small bowel injury

B - Great vessel injury. 1st and/or 2nd rib fractures, as well as scapula and clavicle fractures may cause great vessel (aorta) injury. It is mostly seen in sudden deceleration from MVC and 90% of aortic injuries occur at the **ligamentum arteriosum** which secures the heart to the aorta. (TNCC pgs. 145-146)

19. A discrepancy between blood pressure values and pulse strength, a loud systolic murmur, and mediastinal widening on a chest radiograph are symptoms of which traumatic injury?
    a. Diaphragmatic rupture
    b. Aortic disruption
    c. Traumatic asphyxia
    d. Flail chest

B – Aortic disruption should be considered in severe deceleration injury. S/S include severe chest pain, dyspnea, a loud systolic murmur, blood pressure and pulse strength discrepancies with decreased pulses in lower extremities, and **mediastinal widening** and obscured aortic knob on a chest radiograph. Start large-bore IV's, maintain SBP between 100-120 mmHg, and prepare for surgical repair. (TNCC pg. 158)

20. A patient admitted after a MVC with blunt chest trauma suddenly becomes confused, tachycardic, and hypotensive. You notice jugular vein distension (JVD) and auscultate faint heart sounds. You notice pulsus paradoxus, so you suspect:
    a. Cardiac tamponade
    b. Hypovolemic shock
    c. Cardiogenic shock
    d. Pulmonary embolus

A - Cardiac tamponade. S/S include **Beck's triad** of hypotension, distended neck veins, and muffled heart sounds, **electrical alternans** – alteration of QRS complex amplitude or axis. **pulsus paradoxus** - decrease in stroke volume, SBP (> 10 mm Hg drop during inspiration), and pulse amplitude during inspiration. (TNCC pgs. 157-158)

21. A 28-year-old male with a single stab wound to the left chest just arrived in your level 1 trauma center. VS: HR=130/min, RR=30, BP=78/48 mm Hg. Assessment reveals jugular vein distention and a low ECG amplitude. The experienced trauma nurse would prepare for the following intervention:
    a. Pericardiocentesis
    b. Surgical pericardiectomy
    c. Needle decompression at the 2nd ICS, MCL
    d. Chest tube placement

B - Surgical pericardiectomy (pericardial window). For an unstable patient, the treatment of choice in a trauma center is **surgical repair** or resuscitative thoracotomy, to prevent blood from accumulating in the pericardial sac. Pericardiocentesis is only a temporary solution. (TNCC pg. 158)

22. Resuscitative thoracotomy is most successful in treating:
    a. Penetrating injury resulting in pericardial tamponade.
    b. Blunt chest trauma resulting in hemothorax.
    c. Out-of-hospital cardiac arrest.
    d. Coexistent head trauma.

A – Resuscitative thoracotomy may be necessary when a patient with **penetrating trauma** resulting in pericardial tamponade in a level 1 or 2 center. Anticipate a **pericardiocentesis** guided by echocardiogram if you are in a rural facility and repeat as needed until transfer. (TNCC pg. 158)

23. Resuscitative Endovascular Balloon Occlusion of Aorta (REBOA) is used correctly when:
    a. The catheter is inserted into the distal thoracic aorta (Zone 1) for traumatic arrest.
    b. The catheter is inserted into the distal abdominal aorta (Zone 4) for intra-abdominal hemorrhage.
    c. The catheter is inserted into the distal thoracic aorta (Zone 1) for severe pelvic hemorrhage.
    d. The catheter is inserted into (Zone 2) for retroperitoneal hemorrhage.

A - The catheter is inserted via the femoral artery into the distal thoracic aorta (Zone 1) for traumatic arrest. The balloon is inflated at Zone 3 for severe pelvic or proximal lower extremity bleed. (TNCC pgs. 149-150)

24. A 20-year-old deer hunter falls from a tree stand 20 feet high striking multiple branches. He is anxious and c/o of severe left flank pain radiating to the left shoulder. VS: HR=132, RR=36, BP=80/40, O_2 sat 89%. Ecchymosis is noted at the left flank and his abdomen has a scaphoid appearance. Peristaltic sounds are audible in the left lower chest. The likely cause of these findings is:
    a. Pulmonary contusion
    b. Tension pneumothorax
    c. Great vessel injury
    d. Ruptured diaphragm

D - Ruptured diaphragm. A ruptured diaphragm leads to the abdominal contents shifting upward into the thoracic cavity. As the abdominal organs move into the thoracic cavity, the lungs, heart, and great vessels are displaced. The patient may present with dyspnea, dysphagia (difficulty swallowing), bowel (peristaltic) sounds in the chest, a **progressively scaphoid abdomen**, and decreased breath sounds on the injured side. **Emergent exploratory laparotomy is indicated to repair the injured diaphragm.** (TNCC pgs. 158-159)

25. A patient runs into the ED saying "Help, I've been cut." His abdomen is open and there is evisceration of abdominal contents. While your team is starting the patients IV access, how should you address the abdominal wounds?
    a. Attempt to place the abdominal contents back into the cavity.
    b. Place a sterile dressing over the intestines.
    c. Irrigate the site and leave the wound open.
    d. Cover the intestines with a petroleum gauze.

B - Place a sterile dressing over the intestines is indicated. Dressing may be saline soaked if small evisceration but may cause hypothermia if large evisceration. (Sheehy, pg. 256)

26. A 9-year-old presents to triage complaining of left shoulder pain. He is pale and diaphoretic, VS: HR=120 bpm, RR=24, BP=100/60. Upon further questioning, the child reports he was hit in the stomach during recess yesterday. Which test does the trauma nurse expect to be performed initially?
    a. Shoulder x-ray
    b. FAST exam
    c. CT of the abdomen
    d. Hemoccult

B - FAST (Focused assessment with sonography for trauma) exam. Hemorrhage within the peritoneal cavity often presents as referred pain to the left shoulder, also known as Kehr's sign. Referred pain to neck is called Saegesser's sign. The ED practitioner will perform a FAST exam since it is quick, accurate, noninvasive, and can be repeated without concern for radiation. (TNCC pg. 180)

27. The American Association for the Surgery of Trauma (AAST) developed a grading system for splenic injuries to guide proper treatment and interventions. What grade splenic injury would involve a laceration of vessels producing devascularization to > 25% of the spleen?
    a. Grade II
    b. Grade III
    c. Grade IV
    d. Grade V

C - Grade IV splenic injury. The spleen is highly vascular, with minimal elasticity and flexibility. The goal of spleen injury is nonoperative management to preserve the immunologic function of the spleen, but a splenectomy is highly likely for a Grade 5 injury, age > 55, and hemodynamic instability. (TNCC pg. 174)

28. Patients who have undergone splenectomy have permanent immunologic impairment and are at risk for infection in the first 2 years post splenectomy. The Center for Disease Control (CDC) recommends the following vaccines be administered within 14 days of splenectomy, **EXCEPT:**
    a. Meningococcal
    b. Pneumococcal
    c. Varicella
    d. Influenza

C – The CDC recommends **meningococcal, pneumococcal, and influenza vaccines**, with the first doses given within 14 days of splenectomy. The patient is educated to seek medical care for minor animal bites, unexplained fever, and prior to traveling to regions with endemic malaria. (TNCC pg. 175)

29. A 17-year-old blunt trauma patient complains of RUQ abdominal pain, and you assess umbilical ecchymosis. VS: HR=120, BP= 96/48. Based on the nurse's knowledge of anatomy and trauma, he/she understands the most likely injured organ is the:
    a. Kidney
    b. Spleen
    c. Bowel
    d. Liver

D – Liver injury. RUQ pain and umbilical ecchymosis (**Cullen's sign**) are suggestive of liver injury. LUQ pain radiating to the shoulder is consistent with a spleen injury. Bowel injuries result in absent bowel sounds and generalized abdominal pain. A key nursing intervention when monitoring a minor liver or spleen injury is to **monitor hemoglobin and hematocrit closely**. (TNCC pgs. 172-173)

30. Air in the mediastinum, subcutaneous emphysema, and food particles in the chest tube are findings seen in which injury?
    a. Esophageal injury
    b. Aortic injury
    c. Open pneumothorax
    d. Ruptured diaphragm

A – Blunt esophageal injury is rare, but suspected with subcutaneous emphysema from concurrent pneumothorax, and esophageal matter in the chest tube. (TNCC pgs. 172-173)

31. A CT scan with IV contrast is ordered on a patient with blunt chest and abdominal injury. Which laboratory value would exclude this diagnostic test?
    a. Creatinine of 3.0 mg/dL
    b. Serum glucose of 240 mg/dL
    c. Troponin of 0.10 ng/mL
    d. Hemoglobin of 7.2 gm/dL

A – Creatinine of 3.0 mg/dL. Normal creatinine levels are approximately 0.5-1.2 mg/dL. An elevated level indicates impaired renal function, which increases the risk of contrast-induced nephropathy. (TNCC pg. 179)

32. Renal pedicle avulsion is described as which grade injury?
    a. Grade 2
    b. Grade 3
    c. Grade 4
    d. Grade 5

D – Renal pedicle injury or a shattered kidney is classified as a grade 5, the most severe. S/S include hematuria, costovertebral angle tenderness, and ecchymosis over the flank. (TNCC pg. 179)

33. After being bucked by a horse several times a 21-year-old male is thrown to the ground. On arrival to the ED, he is complaining of scrotal pain and the urge to urinate. On assessment he is tender in the suprapubic area, and you notice bruising to the scrotum and blood at the urinary meatus. Which diagnosis is most reflective of this patient's presentation?
    a. Open book pelvic fracture
    b. Testicular torsion
    c. Urethral injury
    d. Renal injury

C - Urethral injury is more common in males because the urethra is less protected. They are usually a result of high-energy impact or straddle mechanisms and should be considered with any pelvic fracture. (TNCC pgs. 176-177)

34. In urethral injuries, urinary catheter insertion should be withheld until:
    a. A prostate exam is completed.
    b. BUN and creatinine are verified normal.
    c. A retrograde urethrogram is negative.
    d. The patient voids clear urine.

C – Retrograde urethrograms should be completed prior to insertion of a urinary catheter when urethral injury is suspected. Evaluate for blood at the urethral meatus and gross hematuria. Most injuries require a suprapubic cystostomy. (TNCC pg. 179)

35. A 16-year-old football player is admitted following blunt left flank trauma. One day later, he has a decreased hematocrit level and ecchymosis is noted on the back. A likely cause of these findings is:
    a. Mesenteric injury
    b. Retroperitoneal bleeding
    c. Post-renal failure
    d. Pre-renal failure

B - Retroperitoneal bleeding may be noted, often 24 hours later, as bruising (Grey-Turner Sign). Bleeding into this space is expected with moderate to severe **renal or pancreatic trauma** and generally self-tamponades. **FAST exam is not effective** for assessing retroperitoneal organs. Monitoring **urine output is most important**. (TNCC pg.179)

36. A patient has an abdominal contusion at the level of the lap restraint after a high-speed MVC. An anticipated injury is a/an:
    a. Renal laceration
    b. Bowel rupture
    c. First rib fracture
    d. Aortic dissection

B - Bowel rupture. Hollow organs (bowel, stomach, or bladder) may "pop" in response to "lap belt" injury. S/S: involuntary guarding and rebound tenderness. Concurrent injury includes a **"Chance"** fracture of T12-L2 with "lap belt" injury. (TNCC pg. 171)

37. The trauma nurse is precepting a new nurse to monitor abdominal compartment pressures through bladder pressure readings. Which of the following statements by the preceptee would indicate the need for further instruction?
    a. "The patient needs to be positioned supine."
    b. "The transducer needs to be leveled at the symphysis pubis."
    c. "Instillation of 200 ml of dextrose into the bladder should be performed before the pressure reading is obtained."
    d. "The physician needs to be notified for pressure readings > 20 mm Hg."

C - Instillation of 200 ml of dextrose into the bladder. Do not add more than 50 ml of sterile NS before reading the pressure. Insert an indwelling catheter, level at symphysis pubis with patient in supine position. Normal reading is 12-15 mm Hg, a reading > 20 mmHg may require decompression. (TNCC pgs. 445-446)

38. A 57-year-old female was involved in a high speed, frontal impact MVC. On arrival to the trauma bay, she has a positive FAST exam and unstable vital signs. She is taken emergently to the OR for an exploratory laparotomy. The surgeon repairs a liver laceration and splenic capsule rupture, while the patient receives 28 units of blood products. Three days post-op the ICU nurse notes an intra-abdominal pressure of 32 mm Hg, and the ventilator begins alarming due to high pressure. The trauma nurse should anticipate:
    a. Transfusion of 1 unit of PRBC's
    b. Emergent surgery for abdominal compartment syndrome (ACS)
    c. Emergent splenectomy
    d. Immediate peritoneal dialysis

B - Emergent surgery for ACS. Abdominal compartment syndrome is defined as "sustained intra-abdominal pressure (IAP) exceeding **20 mmHg** associated with new organ dysfunction or failure". **Abdominal perfusion pressure (APP) = MAP-IAP**. ACS typically occurs after abdominal trauma with hemorrhage or in patients who received an excessive amount of volume resuscitation. The vena cava is compressed causing a **decrease in venous return**, cardiac output, and renal function. Those at highest risk are pregnant females, patients with ascites, and **morbidly obese**. Treatment includes **surgical decompression of the abdomen** to prevent bowel ischemia, ARDS, increased ICP, MODS, and death. (TNCC pgs. 445-446)

39. In blunt abdominal trauma which of the following organ injuries commonly goes undetected due to its asymptomatic initial presentation?
    a. Liver
    b. Spleen
    c. Pancreas
    d. Bladder

C - The pancreas gets crushed between the abdominal wall and spinal column so suspect in spinal injury. In penetrating trauma suspect pancreatic injury with duodenal damage (also frequently missed). S/S: abdominal tenderness initially, then epigastric pain radiating to back increasing with rigidity and guarding. Monitor the pancreas through FAST exams, amylase, **lipase**, and glucose. (TNCC pg. 175).

40. Anatomic and physiologic changes in pregnancy can confound the typical assessment findings associated with trauma. Pregnancy increases the risk of the following, **EXCEPT**:
    a. Aspiration
    b. Anemia
    c. Disseminated Intravascular Coagulation (DIC)
    d. Cervical spine injury

D – Not spinal injury. Pregnancy increases the risk of pelvic fracture due to softening and relaxation of the sacral ligaments and pubic symphysis, and this widened gait predisposes the gravid patient to falls. Delayed GI emptying increases the **risk of aspiration**. Increased circulating plasma results in **dilutional anemia**. An increase in fibrinogen levels and clotting factors result in a hypercoagulable state that increases the risk for thromboembolism and **DIC**. (TNCC pgs. 333-334)

41. A 34-week pregnant patient sustained blunt abdominal trauma in an MVC. She is complaining of severe back pain and scant amounts of dark red vaginal bleeding. You assess a rising fundal height, a board-like abdomen, and hypotension. Which of the following interventions is **contraindicated** initially?
    a. Administering high-flow oxygen.
    b. Performing a pelvic exam to assess uterine injuries.
    c. Turn the patient 15 degrees to the side.
    d. Transfusing blood products.

B - Performing a pelvic exam is contraindicated until the ultrasound is completed. High-flow O_2 should be administered since the pregnant patient has a decreased functional residual capacity and less tolerant of hypoxia. The fetus is even more sensitive to hypoxia than the mother. **Position the patient 15°** on left side (**tilt back-board if patient is still boarded**) to displace the gravid uterus from compressing the inferior vena cava, possibly leading to a decrease preload and cardiac output. The most common cause of traumatic fetal demise is **placental abruption**. Depending on the location of the tear there **may not be** visible vaginal blood (dark red). Abruption pain is often described as ripping, tearing back pain. (TNCC pgs. 295-96)

42. A patient who is 36 weeks pregnant comes to the ED after a fall. She is anxious with no obvious injuries on assessment. VS: HR=88 bpm, RR=24, BP=108/76, O_2 sat 99%, and FHT's = 140 bpm. ABG's: pH=7.47, $PaCO_2$=30, HCO_3=20 mEq/L. Based on these results, the nurse anticipates the following course of action:
    a. Prepare to intubate the patient since she is in respiratory alkalosis.
    b. Continue monitoring and turn the patient on her left side.
    c. Place the patient on an non-rebreathing mask mask without oxygen since she is hyperventilating.
    d. Infuse 2 liters of LR for hypotension.

B - Monitor the patient and turn her on her left side to prevent supine vena cava syndrome. Anatomic and physiologic changes during pregnancy include an increasing heart rate by 10-20 bpm, a decrease in BP due to increased hormonal levels, aortocaval compression, a state of **respiratory alkalosis** due to increased respiration. (TNCC pgs. 333-334)

43. A patient arrives at your hospital after a motor vehicle collision (MVC). She was a restrained driver with a frontal impact MVC. She reports that she is pregnant and is having abdominal pain. She is unsure how far along she is, but her fundal height is slightly above the umbilicus. The trauma nurse suspects she is how many weeks pregnant?
    a. 16-20 weeks
    b. 20-24 weeks
    c. 24-28 weeks
    d. 28-32 weeks

B - Approximately 20-24 weeks pregnant. Fundal height is an indicator of gestational age. **The fundus is measured in centimeters from the symphysis pubis to the top of the fundus**. The uterus remains protected by the pelvis until 12 weeks gestation. **By 20 weeks, the uterus is at the level of the umbilicus**. At 34-36 weeks, the uterus reaches the costal margin. **Rising fundal height is seen in abruptio placentae**. (TNCC pg. 341)

44. A patient at 38 weeks gestation arrives via EMS after a high-speed MVC with a pulse of 120 bpm and a blood pressure of 80/40. Continuous fetal monitoring reveals fetal bradycardia. Which of the following increases the risk of uterine rupture?
    a. Frequent sexually transmitted infections
    b. Gestational diabetes
    c. Prior cesarean sections
    d. Induction of labor

C – Prior C-sections increase the risk of uterine rupture. Tearing of the uterus is rare but may occur in patients with extreme compression injury or a history of prior cesarean sections. Uterine rupture is associated with high maternal and fetal mortality. (TNCC pg. 336)

45. A 28-week pregnant female is involved in a roll-over MVC. She is G-2, P-1, with a C-section on previous delivery. You palpate fetal parts over the abdomen, maternal blood pressure is 70 systolic, and fetal heart tones are 90 beats/min. The trauma nurse suspects:
    a. Liver laceration
    b. Uterine rupture
    c. Placenta previa
    d. Abruptio placenta

B - S/S of **uterine rupture** include severe, continual abdominal pain and signs of hypovolemic shock, along with asymmetry of the uterus. You may **palpate fetal extremities** outside the uterus. **Normal FHT 120-160 beats/minute**. Fetal bradycardia is a sign of severe distress. (TNCC pg. 336)

46. A patient arrives at your trauma bay after a low speed MVC. She reports that she is 24 weeks pregnant and having lower abdominal pain. Her FAST exam is negative, and a pelvic exam reveals that her cervix is closed. Fetal heart tones are 140 bpm. Which medication does the nurse expect to administer to stop preterm labor?
    a. Hydralazine
    b. Magnesium sulfate
    c. Diazepam
    d. Rocuronium

B - Magnesium sulfate is a tocolytics (stops contractions). Magnesium sulfate causes hypocalcemia which results in a neuromuscular blockade effect. (TNCC pg. 335)

47. The provider orders a Nitrazine test of perineal fluid leaking from a pregnant victim of interpersonal violence who was punched in the stomach. Nitrazine paper will turn what color in the presence of amniotic fluid?
    a. Blue
    b. Red
    c. Green
    d. Yellow

A - Blue 7.0-7.5. Nitrazine paper can be used to test the vaginal pH to determine the breakage of the amniotic sac. Amniotic fluid is in the pH range of 4.5-7.5 and is more sensitive than litmus paper. The pH of **urine is 4.6-6**. (TNCC pg. 341)

48. Which laboratory tests detect fetal red blood cells in the maternal circulation, indicating hemorrhage of fetal blood through the placenta?
    a. Alpha-fetoprotein (AFP)
    b. Thromboelastogram (TEG)
    c. Reticulocyte count
    d. Kleihauer-Betke (KB) test

D – The KB serum test detects fetal red cells in the maternal circulation, used to predict abruptio placentae. It is important in determining the need to administer **Rh immune globulin** when the mother is Rh negative, and the fetus is Rh positive. (TNCC pg. 342)

C. Extremity and Wound Questions (25 Questions) – 29 Sample Questions

1. A patient with a knee dislocation is ordered q 2-hour neurovascular checks. The ED nurse knows they are assessing for:
    a. Peroneal nerve compression
    b. Plexus injury
    c. Abnormal range of motion
    d. Tibia/fibula involvement

    A - Patients with a dislocated knee require frequent neurovascular checks to assess for potential compromise of the **peroneal nerve compression**. (TNCC pg. 211)

2. A potential complication of delayed reduction of a dislocated knee is:
    a. Necrosis of the femoral head
    b. Sciatic nerve compression
    c. Popliteal artery damage
    d. Osteomyelitis of the tibia/fibula

    C - Reduction of a dislocated knee should not be delayed due to the potential for circulatory compromise of the **popliteal artery.** (TNCC pg. 211)

3. Which mechanism of injury is most likely to result in a hip dislocation?
    a. A patient who suffered a seizure and fell from a standing position.
    b. An MVC victim that had their leg outstretched on the brake pedal at the time of impact.
    c. A diver that has suffered an axial loading injury.
    d. The driver of an ATV that rolled over.

    B - When there is a high-impact collision and the **leg is outstretched**, there is a high probability of a posterior hip dislocation. (TNCC pg. 210)

4. A patient with a hip dislocation is most likely to suffer from which complication:
    a. Avascular necrosis of the femoral head
    b. Popliteal artery damage
    c. Peroneal nerve injury
    d. Tibial nerve and artery compromise

    A - A dislocated hip can result in **avascular necrosis of the femoral head** and sciatic nerve injury without timely reduction. (TNCC pg. 210)

5. The trauma nurse receives a patient after a motorcycle crash. To appropriately assess pelvic stability, the nurse applies:
    a. Gentle pressure inward over the iliac wings and downward over symphysis pubis
    b. Gentle pressure inward and downward over the iliac crest
    c. Firm pressure inward over the iliac crest and downward over symphysis pubis
    d. Firm pressure inward and downward over the iliac crest

    A - Gentle pressure inward over the iliac wings and downward and medially and over symphysis pubis. (TNCC pgs. 177-178)

6. Hemorrhage in pelvic fracture results from disruption of which artery?
    a. Renal artery
    b. Iliac artery
    c. Mesenteric artery
    d. Hepatic artery

B – Pelvic fractures cause hemorrhage from laceration to the **iliac artery.** (TNCC pgs. 177-178)

7. A 16-year-old male riding a jet ski crashes into a pier. On arrival to the trauma bay his vital signs are HR=136, RR=32, and BP=84/62. The patient has a "frog leg" appearance and scrotal swelling. A pelvic film shows an open book pelvic fracture. What is the nurse's priority intervention for this patient?
   a. Apply a pelvic binder.
   b. Place bilateral femoral traction.
   c. Transfuse 1 unit of PRBC.
   d. Check for pelvic stability by rocking the pelvis.

A - Apply a pelvic binder. An open book pelvic fracture is caused by anterior-posterior compression. With the symphysis pubis separated the posterior pelvic venous complex and the **internal iliac artery can hemorrhage**. Internally rotating the lower limbs and stabilizing the pelvis with a binder reduces the pelvic volume; binding the pelvis creates a smaller area to collect blood. The initial intervention is to apply a sheet or **pelvic binder at the level of the greater trochanters of the femur**. After stopping the hemorrhage, the patient should receive balanced resuscitation until taken for surgical repair. (TNCC pg. 178)

8. A patient with a complex right tibia-fibula fracture is six hours post-op from an ORIF and one-compartment fasciotomy. Despite having patient-controlled analgesia for pain control he is complaining of increased pain, and a decreased ability to dorsiflex his right foot. The nurse suspects:
   a. Cauda equina syndrome
   b. An arterial occlusion
   c. A deep vein thrombosis
   d. Compartment syndrome

D - Compartment syndrome. There are 4 lower leg muscle compartments. S/S: **Pain out of proportion to injury is the hallmark sign**. Weak peripheral pulses to pulselessness are late signs. Measure compartment pressure with an intracompartmental monitoring device, normal pressure is < 10 mmHg. TX: initially **keep the limb at level of heart (neutral position)**. Prepare for emergency **fasciotomy** when pressure = > 30 mmHg. (TNCC pgs. 202-210)

9. A hunter falls out of his deer stand landing on his feet and x-rays reveal bilateral calcaneal fractures. What other injuries are commonly associated with this injury?
   a. Median nerve injury and/or brachial artery injury due to FOOSH fracture.
   b. Pulmonary contusion and/or rib fractures.
   c. Femoral neck fracture and/or posterior hip dislocation.
   d. Spine injury and/or tibial plateau fracture.

D - Spine injury and/or tibial plateau fracture. Significant force will be transmitted along the body's long axis. Fracture is seen at the initial point of contact (the heels) then continued up the legs and spine. Median nerve injury and/or brachial artery injury is seen with elbow fracture/dislocation. Pulmonary contusions and/or rib fractures are seen with clavicular or scapular fractures. Femoral neck fracture and/or posterior hip dislocation are seen with femur fracture. (TNCC pg. 197)

10. A 6-year-old who was unrestrained in an MVC arrives in the trauma bay. The child has no sensation from the waist down, but the CT scan shows no injuries. Based on the trauma nurse's knowledge of physiology, he/she understands the most likely explanation for these symptoms is:
   a. Neurogenic shock
   b. SCIWORA
   c. Lumbar Fracture
   d. Attention-seeking behavior.

B - SCIWORA. Spinal Cord Injury without Radiographic Abnormalities is seen more often in children < age 8 because children have incomplete development of the skeleton. **MRI** (not x-ray or CT) shows hemorrhage or edema. TX: spinal immobilization and neurosurgical consult. (TNCC pg. 275)

11. A football player has a tibial fracture. Proper immobilization of a traumatic long bone injury is described as:
    a. Immobilization above the injury only
    b. Immobilization below the injury only
    c. Immobilization at the actual site of the injury
    d. Immobilization above and below the injury

    D - Immobilization above and below the injury to avoid movement of fractured bone, which can increase bleeding and risk of fat emboli. (TNCC pg. 215)

12. A 51-year-old man presents to your emergency department with blood dripping from his hand. He reports that his finger was cut off by a saw at work. After controlling the bleeding, the nurse cares for the amputated finger by:
    a. Placing the severed finger in a cup of ice to preserve the tissue.
    b. Scrubbing the amputated digit to reduce the risk of infection.
    c. Placing the severed finger in the biohazard trash container because it likely cannot be replanted.
    d. Wrapping the amputated part in a moist sterile towel, putting it in a plastic bag and placing it on top of crushed ice.

    D - Wrapping the amputated part in a moistened sterile towel, putting it in a bag and placing it on top of crushed ice. Be careful not to freeze the amputated part. (TNCC pgs. 217-218)

13. After fighting with his brother, a 17-year-old male presents to the emergency department with swelling and tenderness to his right hand. A boxer's fracture involves which bone?
    a. Scaphoid
    b. Metacarpal
    c. Ulna
    d. Radius

    B - Metacarpal. A boxer's fracture is a fracture of the neck of the fourth or fifth metacarpal. This fracture typically occurs when the patient punches an object with his dominant hand. Treatment involves a posterior ulnar splint for 3-4 weeks. A Colles fracture is a fracture of distal radius/ulna bones from fall on an outstretched hand. A scaphoid fracture results in tenderness at the anatomic snuffbox. (Sheehy 8th edition pg. 295)

14. A 28-year-old male sustains a mid-shaft femur fracture during a motorcycle crash. He is admitted to the hospital and later that day he is taken to surgery for surgical fixation of the fracture. The next morning the nurse finds the patient confused, diaphoretic, anxious, and short of breath. A petechial rash is noted on his chest. VS: HR=132, RR=36, BP=128/74, O_2 sat 85%. What does the nurse suspect?
    a. Hypovolemia due to blood loss during surgery
    b. Fat embolism syndrome
    c. Pulmonary contusion
    d. Pulmonary embolism

    B - Fat embolism syndrome. Embolic marrow can become dislodged during the manipulation of long bone fractures. The marrow moves to the lungs causing an obstruction known as a fat embolism. Patients normally present with symptoms **24-72 hours after a long bone fracture** or orthopedic injury. S/S: altered mental status (**restlessness**, agitation), **acute respiratory distress, severe hypoxemia**, and a **petechial rash** to head, neck, anterior thorax, or **axillae**. (TNCC pgs. 205-206 and 442)

15. A 69-year-old female discovered twelve hours after a fall where she fractured her hip has developed rhabdomyolysis. What causes the dark red or brown urine in rhabdomyolysis?
    a. Myoglobinuria is the result of muscle injury, causing dark urine.
    b. Hydroxocobalamin is administered for treatment, breaking down myoglobin into vitamin B 12.
    c. Deferoxamine is administered for treatment, breaking down myoglobin into iron.
    d. Rhabdomyolysis causes disseminated intravascular coagulation, causing hematuria.

A - Rhabdomyolysis is caused by muscle-tissue breakdown causing **myoglobin to release resulting in dark brown (cola or tea-colored) urine**. TX: IV fluid resuscitation to maintain **a urine output of 100–300 mL/hour**. Adding **sodium bicarbonate** to the IVF to alkalinize the urine may enhance myoglobin excretion. (TNCC pgs. 210 and 447)

16. Which of the following lab values would be an expected finding in rhabdomyolysis?
    a. Elevated amylase and lipase.
    b. Elevated bilirubin.
    c. Decreased potassium.
    d. Elevated creatine kinase (CK).

D – CK and potassium will be elevated in rhabdomyolysis. Begin aggressive fluid management and alkalinization to produce **urine output of 100-300 mL/hour** in adults to prevent **acute tubular necrosis**. (TNCC pg. 447)

17. Which wound closure is used for deep wounds left open initially due to risk of infection?
    a. Primary
    b. Secondary
    c. Tertiary
    d. Quaternary

C – Tertiary (delayed primary) closure is used for deep wounds that were initially left open and allowed to granulate due to risk of infection. (TNCC pg. 234)

18. EMS brings in a patient after an explosion 30 minutes ago with a tourniquet above the right knee. The right calf has multiple deep lacerations, but bleeding is controlled currently. Removal of a tourniquet is done:
    a. After 2 hours
    b. When a distal pulse cannot be palpated
    c. At the direction of the surgeon
    d. When capillary refill is prolonged

C – At the direction of surgeon. A tourniquet should be placed just above the wound. If transit time is < one hour, the tourniquet remains in place **until the patient is in the OR**. If ineffective, the tourniquet should be tightened or repositioned. A hemostatic bandage or an additional tourniquet may be required. Allow permissive hypotension to decrease bleeding in amputations. (TNCC pg. 220)

19. EMS transports a patient from a housefire with burns to the face, neck, and chest. The patient has stridor and is coughing up carbonaceous sputum. What is the priority intervention?
    a. Calculate the total surface burn area for fluid resuscitation.
    b. Send blood to lab for a carboxyhemoglobin to assess for carbon monoxide toxicity.
    c. Assess the patient for the odor of bitter almonds to determine cyanide toxicity.
    d. Prepare for immediate intubation.

D – Prepare for **immediate intubation** before complete obstruction occurs. (TNCC pg. 237)

20. Prior to calculating the total body surface area (TBSA), the recommended starting point for fluid resuscitation in an adult with significant burn is:
    a. 250 mL/hour
    b. 375 mL/hour
    c. 500 mL/hour
    d. 750 mL/hour

C – 500 mL/hour is the starting point for fluid resuscitation in ages 14 and older. 250 mL/hour for ages 6-13, and 125 mL/hour for ages 5 and under. Avoid starting vascular access through burned tissue if possible. (TNCC pg. 239)

21. A 100-kg adult presents with extensive partial thickness & full-thickness burns from a housefire, measuring 50% body surface area (BSA) & requires fluid resuscitation. According to American Burn Association (ABA) guidelines, what amount of fluid should the patient receive in the first 8 hours after injury?
   a. 2000 ml
   b. 2500 ml
   c. 5000 ml
   d. 10,000 ml

C - 5000 mL. ABA guidelines require **adults** with burns with > **20% BSA** (partial and/or full thickness) receive fluid resuscitation with LR at **2 ml x kg x % BSA burn**. Ex: 2 ml x 100 kg =200 x 50% burn = 10,000/24 hours; **½ = 5,000 in first 8 hours** and ½ = 5,000 over next 16 hours. Urinary output of 30-50 ml/hour for adults is most important. (TNCC pg. 240)

22. A 6-year-old, 20-kg child presents with 10% superficial, 20% deep partial thickness, and 20% full-thickness burns from an immersion injury. What amount of fluid should be administered in the first 8 hours after injury?
   a. 1200 ml
   b. 1500 ml
   c. 2400 ml
   d. 3000 ml

A – 1200 mL. The fluid formula for children with thermal burns is 3 ml lactated Ringer's solution multiplied by weight in kg's multiplied by percentage TBSA of deep partial and full-thickness (not superficial) burns. Half of the fluid is given in the first 8 hours from the time of the burn injury. 3 x 20 x 40 = 2400. The amount given in the first 8 hours = 1200 mL. Adequacy of fluid resuscitation is measured by **minimum urine output of 1-2 mL/kg/hour**. (TNCC pgs. 240-241)

23. There are three classification zones of burns based on the extent and depth of the injury. Which of the following zones is described as moderately damaged resulting in decreased tissue perfusion and edema?
   a. Zone of hyperemia
   b. Zone of stasis
   c. Zone of coagulation
   d. Zone of ulceration

B - The zone of stasis surrounds the zone of coagulation. The tissue in this area may improve with timely treatment. The zone of coagulation is the most severely damaged. The zone of hyperemia is the outermost area of the burn. (TNCC pg. 238)

24. A female patient arrives at the ED after escaping a house fire. There are no obvious burns, but the patient is confused and complaining of headache and nausea. VS: HR=76, RR=18, BP=130/78, O_2 sat 99% on room air. An NRB is applied at 15 L/min and a carboxyhemoglobin (COHb) level is drawn. The lab calls to report a COHb level of 32. What is the priority nursing intervention for this patient?
   a. Discontinuing the O_2 since the oxygen saturation is 98% and the respiratory rate is WNL.
   b. Oxygen should be delivered at 15 L via non-rebreathing mask until the COHb level is less than 10.
   c. The nurse should prepare for intubation due to mechanism of injury.
   d. An IV should be obtained to give IV steroids to reduce swelling.

B - Deliver oxygen via 15 L NRB until COHb normalizes (<10%). The oxyhemoglobin dissociation curve shifts to the left in CO toxicity, so **hemoglobin holds onto oxygen**, yielding **pulse oximetry unreliable**. All patients exposed to CO should receive **high-flow oxygen** to expedite the separation of CO from the Hgb molecule. Patients with a COHb less than 20% usually do not have symptoms. A COHb of 20-30% may cause headache and nausea. COHb of 30-40% may cause confusion. Patients with a COHb of 40-60% are typically unresponsive, and over 60% may result in death. **Pregnant patients are more likely to need hyperbaric oxygenation to support fetal circulation**. (TNCC pg. 237)

25. Which of the following is an indication for an escharotomy?
    a. Perineal burns due to excessive swelling and risk of infection.
    b. Full thickness burns since they extend into the fascia.
    c. When restrictive movement results in failure to ventilate and/or loss of limb.
    d. When carboxyhemoglobin levels exceed 20%, leading to asphyxia.

C – Prepare for an escharotomy in chest wall and extremity circumferential burns that **create restrictive movement that can result in failure to ventilate and/or loss of limb or life**. (TNCC pgs. 243-244)

26. According to the American Burn Association (ABA) criteria, which of the following findings in a 20-year-old burn patient indicates that the patient should be referred to a burn center?
    a. 2% full thickness burns on the left knee.
    b. Partial thickness burns on the anterior thighs.
    c. 8% partial thickness burns on the anterior chest.
    d. Circumferential superficial burns to the forearms.

A - 2% full thickness burns over the left knee. Others include burns of the face, hands, feet, genitalia, or other major joints. Electrical, chemical, and inhalation burns. Partial-thickness burns > 10% TBSA. (Sheehy 8th edition pg. 326)

27. The treatment plan for hydrofluoric acid exposure includes which medication:
    a. Silvadene
    b. Polyethylene glycol (PEG)
    c. Calcium gluconate
    d. Sodium bicarbonate

C – Irrigate hydrofluoric acid (used in window etching) burns for at least 30 minutes and neutralize the fluoride with **calcium gluconate**. (TNCC pg. 247)

28. What is the priority of care when treating a patient with hot molten tar on his hands?
    a. Contact the burn center.
    b. Cool the molten tar with cold water until it is completely cooled.
    c. Cover hands with a petroleum-based ointment and dress to promote emulsification of the tar.
    d. Physically remove the tar.

B – Stop the burning process by **cooling in water until the tar or asphalt is cool to the touch**. Physical removal is not an emergency. After cooling, adherent tar may be covered with a petroleum-based ointment if advised by the burn center. (TNCC pg. 247)

29. Which of the following statements is **INCORRECT** regarding wound care?
    a. Cleaning wounds with tap water or normal saline is vital in reducing infection.
    b. Irrigate with low-pressure and high-pressure to remove contaminants.
    c. Avoid lidocaine with epinephrine where vasoconstriction can impair distal blood flow.
    d. Shave hair around the wound to lessen the risk of infection.

D – Removal of hair from around the wound should be performed with scissors or clippers. Shaving increases infection, so lubricate the hair with antibacterial ointment to lay hair away from wound edges, or clip hair. **Eyebrows should never be shaved** due to loss of anatomic landmark for repair and uneven hair regrowth. Avoid lidocaine with epinephrine on the fingers, toes, ears, nose, and tip of penis. (TNCC pg. 234)

D. Special Considerations Questions (25 Questions) – 31 Sample Questions

1. The family of a deceased trauma patient just arrived at the ED. To support the family in crisis it is important for the trauma nurse to understand the grieving process. Which of the following is **NOT** included in the stages of grief?
   a. Anger
   b. Depression
   c. Bargaining
   d. Frustration

   D - Frustration. The stages of grief are shock and denial, anger, bargaining, depression, and acceptance. During crisis families look to the staff for support and information about the care of their family members. Appropriate response is **"I can't imagine how painful this must be for you."** TNCC teaches the **RESPOND** mnemonic – **R**eassure, **E**stablish rapport, **S**upport, Plan and manage **P**ain, **O**ffer hope, **N**ever deliver bad news alone, and **D**etermine the patient's needs. (TNCC pgs. 373-374)

2. Your patient was the sole survivor of a MVC a week ago. She is now experiencing flashbacks and night terrors, so the nurse suspects:
   a. Post-traumatic Stress Disorder (PTSD)
   b. Acute Stress Disorder (ASD)
   c. Major Depressive Disorder
   d. Anhedonia

   B – **Acute Stress Disorder (ASD)** is more acute and resolves within 30 days of the trauma, whereas PTSD typically starts 3 months after the traumatic event and lasts > 1 month. Experiencing ASD increases the risk of experiencing PTSD. (TNCC p. 375)

3. A veteran was shot while protecting bystanders during a mass shooting in a park. He has a history of angry outbursts and nightmares since returning from combat. These symptoms are suggestive of which condition?
   a. Delirium tremens
   b. Post-traumatic stress disorder (PTSD)
   c. Panic attack
   d. Acute psychosis

   B - PTSD. Flashbacks, nightmares, insomnia, difficulty concentrating, being easily startled (**hypervigilance**), and loss of interest in previously enjoyed activities are common after a terrifying ordeal. Place in a **low stimulus area** and announce yourself prior to entering room. (TNCC pg. 376)

4. Observation of grief reactions can assist the trauma nurse in caring for the grieving family. Nausea, headache, and sleep disturbances are signs of which expression of grief?
   a. Somatic
   b. Cognitive
   c. Affective
   d. Behavioral

   A - Somatic. Expressions of traumatic grief: Somatic grief reveals itself as physical complaints, nausea, headache, sleep disturbances. Cognitive grief is hopelessness and helplessness. Affective grief is guilt, resentment, depression. Behavioral grief is agitation, fatigue, crying, social isolation. (TNCC pg. 378)

5. An abdominal trauma patient who required extensive surgical intervention is in the ICU. On post-op day four vital signs are: T=38°C (101.4°F), HR=126/min, RR=24/min, BP=88/66. In addition to obtaining a white blood cell (WBC) count, initial diagnostic testing would include:
   a. Serum potassium and sodium
   b. Serum lactate and ABG for pH and base deficit
   c. Urine myoglobin and CK

    d. Thromboelastography (TEG)

B - Serum lactate and ABG for pH and base deficit. Lactate assesses the degree of acidosis and oxygen debt gauging end-organ perfusion. TEG assesses global hemostatic and fibrinolytic function. (TNCC pgs. 102 and 445)

6. Parasympathetic stimulation gives rise to which of the following?
    a. Bronchial constriction
    b. Piloerection
    c. Peripheral vasoconstriction
    d. Diaphoresis

A – Parasympathetic stimulation results in bronchial constriction, and decreased heart rate and contractility. Sympathetic stimulation results in increased heart rate and contractility, peripheral vasoconstriction, increased respiratory rate, piloerection (bristled hairs) and increased renin secretion. (TNCC pg. 192)

7. Which of the following is **INCORRECT** regarding the body's compensatory response to shock?
    a. Epinephrine release causes glycogenolysis to provide glucose to the cells.
    b. Baroreceptors in the carotid sinus and aortic arch sense the decrease in stretching, stimulating the sympathetic nervous system.
    c. Metabolic alkalosis results from anerobic metabolism.
    d. Hypoperfusion of the kidneys triggers them to secrete renin, hastening the production of angiotensin I.

C – Anaerobic metabolism results in buildup of lactic acid, resulting in metabolic acidosis. The other statements are correct. Activation of the sympathetic nervous system triggers the "fight or flight" response, releasing epinephrine and norepinephrine. Pulse pressure narrows, and afterload increases. (TNCC pgs. 93-94)

8. Vasopressor administration is contraindicated in the initial resuscitation of the patient in which type of shock?
    a. Cardiogenic
    b. Neurogenic
    c. Septic
    d. Hypovolemic

D - Hypovolemic shock is first treated by fluid resuscitation. If the patient is not responding to damage control resuscitation a vasopressor may be added. Giving dopamine at the first recognition of hypovolemic shock will increase the compensatory vasoconstriction that is occurring and possibly decrease blood flow. Vasopressors are appropriate therapy in cardiogenic, neurogenic, and septic shock states. (TNCC pg. 97)

9. A 16-year-old motorcycle crash patient is awake and alert but unable to move his arms or legs. VS: HR=50, RR=26 and shallow, BP=84/52, O_2 sat 96% on room air. After oxygen is applied and IV access started, what physiological process requires priority intervention?
    a. Normal circulating blood volume.
    b. Increased sympathetic nervous system function.
    c. Decreased parasympathetic function.
    d. Decreased systemic vascular resistance.

D - Decreased SVR (afterload). This patient is in **neurogenic shock** from spinal cord injury, a form of **distributive shock**. Neurogenic shock is a loss of sympathetic vasomotor function which allows unopposed parasympathetic function. This leads to peripheral vasodilation and bradycardia resulting in decreased tissue and organ perfusion. The most common cause is spinal cord injury at T6 or higher. **S/S of neurogenic shock**: warm, dry, flushed skin below the level of injury, cool clammy skin above the level of injury, bradycardia, hypotension, poikilothermy, and priapism. TX: ventilatory support and **augmenting vascular tone with fluids, Norepinephrine, and inotropes such as Dopamine**. (TNCC pgs. 97-98 and 199)

10. Which of the following disorders would **NOT** cause obstructive shock?
    a. Tension pneumothorax
    b. Blunt cardiac injury
    c. Cardiac tamponade
    d. Massive pulmonary embolism

B – Blunt cardiac injury is the most common cause of traumatic cardiogenic shock. Examples of obstructive shock are tension pneumothorax, cardiac tamponade, massive pulmonary embolus, air embolus, abdominal compartment syndrome, and supine vena cava syndrome. (TNCC pg. 97)

11. Why is calcium replacement necessary in massive transfusion?
    a. Crystalloid solutions dilute serum calcium.
    b. Rapid infusers hemolyze cells, resulting in hypocalcemia.
    c. Most traumas are due to alcohol abuse, and patients with alcoholism are typically hypocalcemic.
    d. The preservative citrate in banked blood chelates calcium, leaving it inactive.

D – Citrate binds with calcium, leaving it inactive. Calcium is essential for clotting, so the patient continues to bleed, worsening hemorrhagic shock. Guide replacement on the patient's serum ionized calcium levels. (TNCC pg. 99)

12. A trauma patient is slightly anxious, with a HR=96, RR=16, and a BP=120/80. Identify the class of hemorrhagic shock.
    a. Class I (10-15% blood loss).
    b. Class II (15-30% blood loss).
    c. Class III (30-40% blood loss).
    d. Class IV (> 40% blood loss).

A - Class I, (10-15 % blood loss). Pulse increases (> 100) and pulse pressure narrows at Class II, BP decreases at Class III, anuria at Class IV. If scenario includes pelvic fracture, expect Class IV – estimated 3000 ml blood loss. (TNCC pg. 96)

13. A 20-year-old multi-trauma patient is undergoing damage control surgery and blood transfusions after a rollover MVC. Which of the following findings is reflective of physiological stabilization?
    a. Respirations of 24 per minute.
    b. Heart rate of 120 per minute.
    c. Systolic blood pressure of 78 mm Hg.
    d. Urine output of 0.5-1 ml kg per hour.

D - Normal urinary output is 0.5-1.0 ml/kg/hour for adults and 1-2 ml/kg/hour in a pediatric patient. Urinary output is the best measurement of normalizing organ perfusion and cardiac output. RR of 24 likely indicates an acidotic state related to hypoperfusion. HR of 120 shows continued compensation for low cardiac output and hypoperfusion. Hypotension indicates uncompensated shock. (TNCC pg. 104)

14. A 2-year-old child presents to your rural emergency department after injury from an automobile versus pedestrian injury. Two 20 ml/kg isotonic crystalloid boluses are infused with no improvement in blood pressure. While awaiting transport to a trauma center, what intervention would the nurse next anticipate:
    a. Infusion of IV Dopamine to increase blood pressure.
    b. Infusion of blood products at 10 ml/kg.
    c. Infusion of blood products at 20 ml/kg.
    d. Open thoracotomy since survivability is low.

B – Blood products at 10ml/kg after 2 crystalloid fluid boluses at 20 ml/kg and there is no improvement. Dopamine would only be started only after adequate balanced resuscitation. (TNCC pg. 238)

15. A 78-year-old MVC patient arrives in the trauma bay after a prolonged extrication. His HR is 52, BP is 68/palpation, and he is unresponsive to pain despite blood administration. This patient is likely in which phase of shock?
    a. Compensated shock
    b. Decompensated shock
    c. Irreversible (refractory) shock
    d. Progressive shock

C - Irreversible (refractory) shock. S/S of irreversible shock are unresponsiveness, bradycardia, marked hypotension, shallow respirations, clammy skin, severe acidosis, and coagulopathies. There are 3 stages of shock – compensated (BP stable), decompensated or progressive (hypotension), and irreversible (bradycardia). (TNCC pgs. 92-93)

16. An unrestrained roll-over MVC patient presents with abdominal tenderness and distension. Vital signs: BP=74/50, HR=140, RR=40. Based on the trauma nurse's knowledge, what intervention is anticipated?
    a. 3 liters of warmed isotonic crystalloids.
    b. 2 liters of warmed crystalloids and 2 units warmed packed RBC's.
    c. 4 units warmed PRBC's, 4 units FFP, equal volume of platelets.
    d. 1 unit of warmed PRBC's and 2 units FFP.

C - Start with 4 units of blood, FFP, platelets. This patient is in acute hypovolemic shock from blood loss and requires a massive transfusion at **1:1:1 of PRBC's, FFP, and platelets.** Electrolyte abnormalities after massive resuscitation include **hypocalcemia,** hypomagnesemia, and potassium irregularities. Transfuse O negative pRBC's in females of child-bearing age, O positive in males and postmenopausal women. (TNCC pg. 99)

17. What is the major benefit of hypotensive resuscitation in a bleeding patient?
    a. Reducing the risk of hypothermia from blood transfusions
    b. Reducing the risk of transfusion related acute lung injury (TRALI)
    c. Limiting blood loss by allowing SBP of 70-80 mm Hg
    d. A balanced resuscitation limits hyperchloremic metabolic acidosis

C - Limiting blood loss by allowing SBP 70-80 mm Hg. The goal of **permissive hypotension** is maintaining SBP 70-80 prior to surgery, then "plugging the holes" via **damage control surgery**. Increased blood pressure increases intravascular hydrostatic pressure, worsening blood loss in a bleeding patient. The risk of permissive hypotension is organ hypoperfusion. Permissive hypotension is contraindicated in head trauma. (TNCC pg. 98)

18. A 27-year-old male was ejected from a car at 70 mph. He presents to the trauma bay in spinal immobilization, is intubated, and has two large-bore IV lines in place. His abdomen is rapidly distending. VS: HR=140, RR=12, BP=74/50, O_2 sat= 92%. The priority of care is:
    a. Obtaining a computed tomography (CT) scan to rule over liver injury.
    b. Rapid infusion of 2 liters of warmed crystalloids.
    c. 1 unit of packed RBCs to increase blood pressure.
    d. Damage control surgery to control hemorrhage.

D - Damage control surgery to control hemorrhage. Rapid fluid resuscitation prior to surgery will worsen hypothermia, metabolic acidosis, and coagulopathy (the lethal triad of trauma). Current standards refer to the "lethal diamond", adding hypocalcemia. (TNCC pg. 98)

19. Five days post injury a 58-year-old mechanically ventilated, multi-trauma STICU patient has the following vital signs: HR=132, BP=78/40. Pulmonary artery readings reveal CVP=5, PAOP=19, SVR=1690, CI=2.0. Urine output has been 15 ml/hour for the last 2 hours. Skin is cool and mottled, and the pulse oximeter is not sensing. These findings suggest:
    a. Hypovolemic shock
    b. Cardiogenic shock
    c. Brain herniation
    d. Early sepsis

B - Cardiogenic shock can develop as part of MODS. Right heart pressure (CVP – central venous pressure) is normal, but the left pressure (PAOP – pulmonary artery occlusive pressure) is high due to left ventricular dysfunction. SVR (systemic vascular resistance) is elevated, and CI (cardiac index) is low. These vital signs may be seen in late sepsis, but not in early sepsis. (TNCC pg. 97)

20. You are working at a level 1 trauma center. The attending physician orders a TEG test on an unhelmeted motorcycle crash patient with a scalp laceration, chest wall ecchymosis, and bilateral femur fractures. His vital signs are as follows: HR=112, RR=22, BP=105/68. What is the purpose of using a thromboelastography (TEG) test?
    a. It is an isoenzyme to diagnose cardiac contusion.
    b. TEG detects intracranial bleeding early.
    c. It predicts the need for transfusion and guides transfusion strategy.
    d. TEG detects fat emboli after long bone fractures.

C - TEG guides transfusion strategy. Viscoelastic testing TEG, TEM, and ROTEM are point-of-care tests to evaluate clot formation and strength, platelet function, fibrinolysis, and coagulation. These tests are useful in guiding transfusion strategy. (TNCC pg. 104)

21. Why are children at higher risk for hypoglycemia?
    a. Metabolic demands are higher than adults, and glycogen stores are limited.
    b. Children have a lower blood glucose due to increased exercise.
    c. Children have a higher incidence of eating disorders.
    d. Children ingest more water, diluting blood glucose.

A – Children have a higher metabolic rate and limited glycogen stores. Hypoglycemia decreases the level of consciousness and may cause seizures. (TNCC pg. 280)

22. Selection of the provider with the most experience in difficult airway management is recommended in intubation of the bariatric patient. Which position is preferred for better visualization of the pharyngeal landmarks?
    a. Trendelenburg
    b. High fowlers
    c. Ramped
    d. Semi fowlers

C – A **ramped position with the head elevated**, with the external auditory canal parallel with the sternal notch, allows for better visualization of the pharyngeal landmarks in bariatric patients. Blankets can be used to elevate the head and torso into position. (TNCC pg. 303)

23. Why is insertion of a gastric tube important after intubating the pediatric patient?
    a. Crying and bag-mask ventilation cause swallowed air and gastric distention.
    b. Children use their abdominal muscles for breathing.
    c. Pediatric patients are at a higher risk for developing an ileus.
    d. The abdominal organs are less protected by the rib cage.

A – Crying and positive-pressure ventilation cause children to swallow air, leading to gastric distention. Gastric distention can interfere with adequate respiration so insert a gastric tube after intubation. (TNCC pg. 280)

24. Why is the use of computerized tomography (CT) scans for head trauma limited in children, especially those less than 5 years of age?
    a. The PECARN study shows CT scans are not recommended for children with traumatic brain injury.
    b. CT scans are erroneous in pediatrics, MRIs should be ordered for accuracy.
    c. Focused assessment sonography for trauma (FAST) exams are more accurate than CT scans in pediatrics.
    d. Ionizing radiation exposure is linked to an increased risk of leukemia and solid-organ malignancies.

D – Research shows that ionizing radiation exposure via CT scanners correlates with an increased lifelong **risk of leukemia and solid-tumor cancers**. Children 0-5 years of age are most susceptible to radiation. (TNCC pg. 283)

25. A victim of assault is pronounced dead after a prolonged resuscitation attempt. Which of the following should be performed while the nurse prepares the body for the medical examiner?
    a. Dry and store each item of patient clothing in a separate paper bag.
    b. Clean the body with hydrogen peroxide.
    c. Remove all tubes and lines so the family does not see them.
    d. Place plastic bags over the patient's hands.

A - Dry and store each item of patient clothing in a separate paper bag. The body should **not** be washed as there may be additional collection of evidence. All tubes and lines should be left in place for a medical examiner's case. Store forensic evidence in **paper, not plastic.** Do not dry evidence with heat. (TNCC pgs. 367-368)

26. The nurse notices a bullet fragment on the stretcher after transporting a patient with a gunshot wound to surgery. Proper evidence collection includes:
    a. Comparing it to the size of holes in his clothes.
    b. Placing the bullet fragment in a sealed and labeled container or envelope.
    c. Sending the fragment to pathology for analysis.
    d. Photographing the fragment and noting it in the record.

B - Placing the bullet fragment in a sealed and labeled container or envelope. The chain-of-custody for potential evidence requires that it be within the possession of the healthcare professional who initially discovered it and handled as little as possible. Chain-of-custody **ensures the integrity of the evidence**. Document the law enforcement officer's name, agency, and badge number. (TNCC pgs. 367-368)

Forensic Evidence Collection

- Do not cut through tears, rips, holes or stains when removing clothing.
- Place all evidence in **paper bags** or cardboard boxes, do not use **plastic for risk of molding from moisture**.
- Place **paper bags** over the patient's hands if suspected recent discharge of a firing arm.
- Do **NOT** label wounds as entrance and exit wounds.
- Use sterile gloved hand or metal forceps with rubber tips to remove metal projectiles.
- Preserve paint chips from car versus pedestrian for forensic matching.
- Document law enforcement agency, officer's name, and badge number who received evidence.

27. Elder abuse is underreported due to the following reasons, **EXCEPT**:
    a. Reliance on the caregiver.
    b. Retaliation by the caregiver.
    c. Feelings of shame and embarrassment.
    d. The abuser is unknown to the victim.

D – Most elder abuse occurs in the home by a caregiver who is the spouse or adult child. The victim fears retribution, losing their home, or isolation. (TNCC pg. 354 and Sheehy 8th edition pg. 510)

28. In interpersonal violence, what is reported as the most prognostic factor of future death?
    a. Spiral fracture of the humerus.
    b. Strangulation.
    c. Burns with lines of demarcation.
    d. Sexual abuse.

B – Strangulation is a severe act of violence used to show power and control over the victim. Strangulation is correlated to a 7.5-fold increased risk of homicide. (TNCC pgs. 351 and 358)

29. Which of the following statements is **CORRECT** when inserting an oropharyngeal airway (OPA) in a child?
    a. Depress the tongue using rigid suction and insert the OPA at a 90-degree angle, then turn.
    b. Measure the correct size airway by placing the proximal end at the tip of the child's nose to the tip of the earlobe.
    c. Use a tongue blade and direct insertion technique with the oral airway curving downward.
    d. Oropharyngeal airways should not be used in pediatric patients.

C – Use a direct insertion technique with the oral airway curving downward to avoid damage to the soft palate and to limit the potential for subsequent bleeding. (TNCC pg. 275)

30. Which of the following statements is **INCORRECT** regarding burn trauma in pediatric patients?
    a. The modified Lund and Browder chart is considered the most accurate method for calculating burn size.
    b. The patient's palm from the crease of the wrist to the fingers is roughly equivalent to 1%.
    c. Prior to calculating the TBSA, the recommended starting point for fluid resuscitation is 250 mL/hour for 6-13 years of age.
    d. The burn formula for children with thermal burn is 4 ml x weight in kg x %TBSA for 24-hour fluid requirement.

D – The fluid formula for children with a thermal burn is 3 mL x weight in kg x % TBSA for 24-hour fluid requirement. (TNCC pgs. 239 and 245)

31. Which of the following statements is **INCORRECT** regarding the geriatric trauma patient?
    a. Falls in this patient population are primarily low-energy events and occur from a standing height or lower.
    b. The most common injuries resulting from falls in the older adult are lacerations, traumatic brain injury, and fractures, especially of the hip.
    c. Isotonic fluids and blood products should be utilized to achieve a systolic BP of 90 mm Hg in head trauma.
    d. A heart rate of greater than 90 bpm may indicate significant physiologic stress in the older adult.

C – Avoid hypotension in patients with head trauma, keep **systolic blood pressure 100 to 110 mm Hg in older adults**. (TNCC pg. 322)

E. Continuum of Care Questions (15 Questions) – 17 Sample Questions

1. It is important for the trauma nurse to understand injury prevention and control. The "3 E's" of injury prevention are:
   a. Engineering, enforcement, and education
   b. Experience, epidemiology, and etiology
   c. Empowerment, encouragement, and exploration
   d. Examination, evaluation, and extrapolation

   A - Engineering, enforcement, and education. The "4 E's" of injury prevention are engineering (technology), enforcement (legislation), education, & economic incentives. (TNCC pg. 4)

2. The Haddon Injury Matrix is the most widely used model of injury prevention. Installing pool fencing is an example of which phase of injury prevention?
   a. Primary
   b. Secondary
   c. Tertiary
   d. Quaternary

   A – Primary injury prevention aims to eliminate the occurrence of the injury and includes installing fencing around pools to prevent drowning. (TNCC pg. 4)

3. Advocating for speed humps and/or bumps in a community is an example of what phase of injury prevention?
   a. Primary
   b. Secondary
   c. Tertiary
   d. Quaternary

   A – Primary injury prevention aims to eliminate occurrence of the injury, and includes **speed humps/bumps**, DUI check points, stoplights at dangerous intersections. (TNCC pg. 4)

4. Secondary injury prevention seeks to:
   a. Prevent the occurrence of the injury.
   b. Reduce the severity of the injury.
   c. Improve the outcomes related to the injury.
   d. Analyze injury risk factors.

   B - Reduce the severity of the injury. **Secondary** prevention aims to reduce the severity of the injury and includes **air bags** and restraints. **Tertiary** prevention's goal is to reduce the consequences and improve the outcomes related to the injury and includes utilizing evidence-based practice. (TNCC pg. 4)

5. The following are examples of secondary injury-prevention strategies, **EXCEPT**:
   a. Seat belts
   b. Car seats
   c. DUI checkpoints
   d. Helmets

   C – Secondary phase of injury prevention focuses on the reduction in the severity of the injury that has occurred. Examples include seat belts, air bags, car seats, and helmets. **DUI checkpoints prevent MVC's**, so are primary injury prevention. (TNCC pg. 4)

6. Key elements of an effective injury prevention program include the following, **EXCEPT**:
   a. Identify the primary causes of injury and death in the community.
   b. Develop your own prevention programs to be a leader in injury prevention. Do not use preexisting programs.
   c. Embrace the media for opportunities to educate.
   d. Work with elected leaders to create effective laws promoting prevention.

B - You should work with preexisting programs, media, and elected officials after identifying causes of injury in your community. (ACS *Resources for Optimal Care of the Injured Patient 2022* pgs. 20-21)

7. Multiple trauma patients arrive after a mass shooting in a nightclub. The purpose of the "Across the Room" observation during the initial trauma assessment allows the nurse to:
   a. Rapidly assess for internal bleeding.
   b. Re-prioritize circulation before airway and breathing.
   c. Appropriately triage the injury.
   d. Promptly activate the trauma team.

   B - to re-prioritize circulation before airway and breathing. Rapid identification and treatment are paramount and takes precedence over airway or breathing. (TNCC pg. 42)

8. A hunter that fell from a deer stand is brought to your rural emergency department in the back of a pick-up truck complaining of paralysis. The transfer process from the rural facility to a trauma center should be initiated:
   a. After the required surgeries to stabilize the patient.
   b. After all diagnostic tests are completed.
   c. When stabilization efforts are in process, and it is identified that the patient's needs exceed the facilities resources.
   d. After the primary and secondary assessments are completed, so all injuries are identified.

   C - When stabilization efforts are in process, and it is identified the patient's needs exceed the facilities resources. (TNCC pg. 380)

9. A patient involved in an MVC is being stabilized at a rural facility. Which injury would mandate transfer of the patient to a trauma center?
   a. Spinal cord deficit
   b. Radial artery injury
   c. Glasgow Coma Score of 14
   d. Non-displaced skull fracture

   A - Spinal cord deficit. Criteria for transfer to a Level 1 or 2 trauma center: penetrating injury or open skull fracture, GCS <14 or lateralizing neurologic signs, Spinal fracture, or spinal cord deficit, >2 unilateral rib fractures with pulmonary contusion, open long bone fracture, and/or significant torso injury with advanced co-morbidity disease (renal disease, coronary artery disease, COPD, and diabetes) **Go to closest trauma center that has the required resources.** (TNCC pg. 428)

10. With no air transport available, and based on the CDC Field Triage Guide, a 35-year-old who fell from a third-floor balcony should be transported to a:
    a. Level I trauma center that is two hours away.
    b. Level II trauma center 45 minutes away.
    c. Level III hospital 20 minutes away.
    d. Critical-access hospital 10 minutes away.

    B – Adults who fall > 20 feet (one story is equal to 10 feet) or children who fall > 10 feet should be "transported to a trauma center, which depending upon the defined trauma system, need not be the highest-level trauma center". (TNCC pgs. 15 and 426)

11. The second collision that occurs during an MVC is when:
    a. The vehicle hits another object.
    b. Internal organ structures collide within the body cavity.
    c. The vehicle occupant collides with the vehicle interior.
    d. Internal organs meet the resistance of supporting structures.

    C – When the vehicle occupant collides with the interior of the vehicle. 1st Impact - vehicle hits another object. 2nd impact - vehicle occupant collides with the vehicle interior. 3rd impact - internal organ structures collide within the body cavity and internal organs meet the resistance of supporting structures – **tear of ligamentum arteriosum from shearing forces**. (TNCC pg. 28)

12. Injuries that commonly result during a driver's side lateral impact (T-bone) are:
    a. Clavicle and left rib fractures
    b. Neck extension & flexion injury
    c. Crushing pelvic injury
    d. Sternal blunt injury

A - Clavicle and left ribs. Lateral impact injury patterns depend on where the individual is in the vehicle in relation to the impact. Potential injuries in lateral impact are the aorta, clavicle, lateral pelvic and abdominal, and lateral head, and neck. (TNCC pgs. 29-30)

13. While caring for a gunshot wound patient, the trauma nurse recognizes that:
    a. Handguns are a high velocity weapon.
    b. Shotguns are medium velocity weapons.
    c. Low velocity wounds are the most complex.
    d. Velocity holds the greatest potential for injury.

D - Velocity holds the greatest potential for injury. High velocity wounds are more complex than low velocity wounds (stab wound) because of the greater velocity energy and the cavitation forces. (TNCC pg. 33)

14. A severely injured child is transported to the ED in cardiac arrest. To best facilitate the family's understanding of the event the nurse should:
    a. Arrange for the ED nurse manager to speak with the family members.
    b. Arrange for the parents to be at the bedside.
    c. Place the family in the family room.
    d. Call the hospital chaplain to remain with the family in the family waiting room.

B - Arrange for the parents to be at the bedside. Current research shows most family members want to be present during the resuscitation of a loved one. ENA supports the concept of family presence and believes that it should be offered when possible. Family presence during resuscitation assists in the grieving process, provides closure for survivors, and reduces questioning if personnel were adequately attempting resuscitation. (TNCC pg. 379)

15. Rehabilitation for the trauma patient begins after:
    a. Stabilization
    b. Transfer to ICU
    c. Entering the rehabilitation unit
    d. Surgery

A - After stabilization. (ACS *Resources for Optimal Care of the Injured Patient 2022* pgs. 105-106)

16. Speech therapy, occupational therapy, and physical therapy are vital parts of the rehabilitation team. Which therapist's role is to restore the patient's ability to complete daily tasks such as cooking and bathing?
    a. Speech therapy
    b. Occupational therapy
    c. Physical therapy
    d. Psychologist

B – Occupational therapy works with the patient to regain the ability to perform daily tasks. Speech therapy assists with communication and swallowing. Physical therapy improves movement and function through stretching and exercises.

17. A 28-year-old with a history of depression dies in the emergency department from a self-inflicted gunshot wound to the head. Who is the best person to approach the family about possible organ donation?
    a. The trauma surgeon who informed the family about the death.
    b. The trauma program manager.
    c. Organ procurement representative.
    d. The emergency nurse who is supporting the family.

    C – The person who approaches the family about donation must be a **trained requester or local organ procurement representative**. Early notification gives the OPO representative adequate time to prepare the family for the request to donate a loved one's orans or tissue. (Sheehy pg. 448)

F. Professional Issues (15 Questions) – 22 Sample Questions

1. The primary responsibility of a trauma center's Performance Improvement and Patient Safety (PIPS) program is to:
    a. Monitor and continually improve structures, processes, and outcomes within the institution.
    b. Track trauma surgeon response times.
    c. Monitor trauma center diversion statistics.
    d. Examine delays in operating room availability.

    A - Monitor and continually improve processes and outcomes. Trauma PI is multidisciplinary, with a feedback loop. (TNCC pg. 20 and ACS *Resources for Optimal Care of the Injured Patient 2022* pgs. 119-120)

2. Which level of performance improvement (PI) event review is conducted by an in-house multi-disciplinary committee after a mortality or sentinel event?
    a. Primary
    b. Secondary
    c. Tertiary
    d. Quaternary

    C – **Tertiary review** is conducted by a multidisciplinary committee after mortalities or sentinel events. Primary review is conducted by the PI coordinator. Secondary review is when the primary reviewer sends the case for physician review. (ACS *Resources for Optimal Care of the Injured 2022* pgs. 119-120)

3. This PI review may be provided by an outside agency after the death of a pediatric patient in a low-volume adult trauma facility.
    a. Primary
    b. Secondary
    c. Tertiary
    d. Quaternary

    D – **Quaternary review** may be needed when there is no loop closure in the primary, secondary, or tertiary performance improvement (PI) review. (ACS *Resources for Optimal Care of the Injured 2022* pgs. 119-120)

4. The American College of Surgeons (ACS) provides the following, **EXCEPT**:
    a. Provides objective, external review of the resources needed for high-quality trauma care.
    b. Validates that a hospital is performing as a trauma center and meets the criteria contained in *Resources for Optimal Care of the Injured Patient.*
    c. Designates trauma facilities through their regulatory governmental authority.
    d. Performs on-site facility reviews by a peer review team experienced in trauma care.

    C - ACS does NOT designate trauma centers but validates that the hospital meets the criteria. (ACS *Resources for Optimal Care of the Injured Patient*)

5. A trauma center's designation level is a measure of:
    a. Staff members' commitment to patient care.
    b. A trauma center's OR and bed capacity.
    c. Clinical resources available to care for trauma patients.
    d. Compliance with The Joint Commission trauma standards.

C - Clinical resources available to care for trauma patients. (ACS *Resources for Optimal Care of the Injured Patient*)

6. The primary goal of providing feedback to referring facilities is to:
    a. Increase the number of referrals from outlying hospitals.
    b. Decrease the number trauma referrals deemed medically unnecessary.
    c. Meet HIPAA requirements for information portability.
    d. Improve the process of care and future patient outcomes.

D - Improve the process of care and future patient outcomes. (ACS *Resources for Optimal Care of the Injured Patient*)

7. What is the formal peer-review process for reviewing trauma deaths and complications on a regular basis?
    a. Mortality and morbidity (M & M)
    b. Root cause analysis
    c. Sentinel event
    d. Audit

A - Mortality and morbidity reviews focus on improving the process. These peer-reviewed meetings are an opportunity to examine unexpected outcomes to identify system or process deficits, knowledge shortcomings, and errors in clinician judgment. The process does not lay blame, and in fact. is legally protected from any future litigation. (ACS *Resources for Optimal Care of the Injured Patient*)

8. Minimum criteria for full trauma team activation include the following, **EXCEPT**:
    a. Confirmed BP < 90 mm Hg at any time during transport.
    b. Gunshot wound (GSW) to extremity distal to elbow or knee.
    c. GCS score < 9 with mechanism attributed to trauma.
    d. Emergency physician's discretion.

B - GSW that is proximal, not distal meets minimum criteria. (ACS *Resources for Optimal Care of the Injured Patient*)

9. A patient requires transfer from a level 4 facility to a level 2 trauma center. Prior to transport, an accepting physician must accept the patient. By meeting this requirement, the hospital is complying with:
    a. The Joint Commission recommendations
    b. EMTALA standards
    c. Centers for Medicare and Medicaid Services mandate (CMS)
    d. American College of Surgeons' (ACS) requirements

B - EMTALA standards under federal COBRA laws. Medical screening and stabilization, informed consent, accepting physician, and appropriate transport are the responsibilities of the transferring facility. (TNCC pg. 427)

10. The National Incident Management System (NIMS) requires that hospitals have plans and procedures in place to be prepared for emergency situations, such as mass casualty incidents and disasters. A system that creates a hospital command structure is which of the following?
    a. Federal Emergency Management Agency (FEMA)
    b. Hospital Incident Command System (HICS)
    c. American Red Cross

d. Disaster Medical Assistance Team (DMAT)

B - HICS is NIMS approved for hospitals to use in mass casualty incident response. It provides a command structure with specific job functions under each command level. (Sheehy 8th edition pg. 37)

11. What stage of disaster management is the act of stockpiling supplies?
    a. Mitigation
    b. Preparedness
    c. Response
    d. Recovery

B - Preparedness is stockpiling, practicing disaster drills, and developing mutual aid agreements. Mitigation is the act of performing a hazardous vulnerability assessment. Response is disaster triage and treating patients. Recovery is replenishing supplies, disposing of wastes, and psychosocial care. (TNCC pgs. 394-395)

12. During disaster triage a patient is determined to be salvageable but requires immediate intervention to survive. What color tag would be used for this patient?
    a. Green
    b. Yellow
    c. Red
    d. Black

C - Red (immediate) are first transported to the highest level of care. Priority determinations are made based on a color-coded triage system, such as the **START** Disaster triage. START (Adult) = **"30, 2, can do"** based on **RPM (respiration, perfusion, mental status**). (TNCC pg. 409)

13. After an airplane crash, a patient is unable to ambulate, has a respiratory rate of 20 breaths/minute, a capillary refill less than 2 seconds, and follows commands. Using mass casualty START triage for adults, this patient is classified as:
    a. Green
    b. Yellow
    c. Red
    d. Black

B – Yellow. START triage is based on RPM, respiration, perfusion, and mental status at 30-2-can do. This patient is unable to ambulate so not green, but everything else is OK so he is delayed (yellow). (TNCC pg. 409)

14. A plane just crashed near your facility and your rural hospital will be receiving multiple patients. A disaster has been called but you have only 4 ED nurses onsite. Which of the following patients is the highest priority?
    a. A 20-year-old with an obvious upper thigh deformity, but pulses intact. RR=20, cap refill < 2 secs, following commands.
    b. A minimally responsive 40-year-old, pale, with shallow respirations of 34.
    c. A 6-year-old ambulatory male, who is crying and has with dried blood on his forehead.
    d. An unresponsive, apneic, pulseless 16-year-old male.

B - A minimally responsive adult with respirations > **30**. Priority determinations are made based on a color-coded triage system, such as the **START** Disaster triage. START (Adult) = **"30, 2, can do"** based on **RPM (respiration, perfusion, mental status**). **Jump START (Pediatric)** includes 5 positive pressure breaths prior to tagging black. (TNCC pg. 409)

15. A chemical spill from an overturned tanker truck occurred at your local factory and multiple patients will require treatment. Decontamination principles require that:
    a. The hot zone is established at the hospital.
    b. The warm zone is a minor medical treatment area.
    c. The cool zone is established at the scene.
    d. The cold zone is a treatment area free from contamination.

D - The cold zone is a treatment area free from contamination. Hot zone: established where the contamination occurred; medical TX is only for life-threatening emergencies by providers in protective garments. **Warm zone**: active decontamination with soap and water. **Cold zone**: treatment area free from contamination. **Set up the decontamination tent opposite of wind.** (TNCC pg. 403)

16. Migrant workers accidentally sprayed with pesticides present to the emergency department entrance with excessive tearing, salivation, and respiratory secretions. What is the nurse's first action?
    a. Don your personal protective equipment and decontaminate the patients.
    b. Administer 2 to 5 mg of Atropine IV, repeated every 3 to 5 minutes.
    c. Prepare for immediate intubation and mechanical ventilation.
    d. Administer pralidoxime (protopam chloride 2-PAM) IV.

A – The priority intervention is to **don full personal protective equipment**, including gloves and goggles. The patient's clothing and vomitus must be handled with caution and disposed of carefully. **Atropine and 2-PAM** are administered along with 100% oxygen, and possible intubation. (TNCC pgs. 402 and 418)

17. You are caring for a patient who was onsite when a radiological dispersal device detonated. The nurse anticipates the patient to experience what symptoms?
    a. Body aches
    b. Shortness of breath
    c. GI bleeding
    d. Hearing loss

C - GI symptoms such as nausea, vomiting and GI bleeding are some of the first symptoms of radiation exposure. Practice **time, distancing, and shielding** to reduce risk of radiation. (TNCC pg. 404)

18. EMS transports a patient to the emergency department with a fragment of machinery in his thigh after a factory explosion. His injury is an example of which type of blast injury:
    a. Primary blast injury
    b. Secondary blast injury
    c. Tertiary blast injury
    d. Quaternary blast injury

B – Flying debris and other projectiles causing impalements, fractures, and amputations **secondary to the explosion**. **Pneumothorax**, concussions, ruptured tympanic membranes, etc. occur from the primary blast. (TNCC pgs. 34-35)

19. Burnout symptoms are organized into categories based on symptoms. Decreased job satisfaction and absenteeism is classified under which category?
    a. Decreased sense of personal accomplishment.
    b. Emotional exhaustion.
    c. Physical exhaustion.
    d. Depersonalization.

A – Burnout occurs gradually, and is organized into three categories, emotional exhaustion, depersonalization, and decreased sense of accomplishment. Absenteeism, frustration, decreased satisfaction with the job, and thinking about quitting are categorized under **decreased sense of accomplishment**. Headaches and sleep disturbances are categorized as emotional exhaustion. Sadness is under depersonalization. (TNCC pgs. 383-384)

20. Which of the following would be a violation of the Health Information Portability and Accountability Act (HIPAA)?
    a. Sharing patient information between healthcare providers.
    b. A nurse accessing the records of a family member the next day.
    c. Using a de-identified x-ray for educational purposes without patient consent.
    d. Giving patient information to poison control.

B - A nurse accessing the records of a family member the next day. The goal of HIPAA is to assure that individuals' health information is properly protected while allowing the flow of health information needed to provide and promote high quality health care. (Sheehy 8th edition pg. 5)

21. Massive bleeding can result from many types of injuries and victims can die within 5 to 10 minutes if nothing is done. What is the **FIRST** step of the "Stop the Bleed" program?
    a. Be aware of your surroundings and call 911.
    b. Locate life-threatening injury.
    c. Engage direct and steady pressure with both hands.
    d. Elevate the extremity above the level of the heart.

A – The mnemonic **BLEED lists the steps of "Stop the Bleed." B - Be aware of your surroundings and call 911**. L – Locate life-threatening injury and expose the bleeding. E – Engage direct pressure. E – Elevate the extremity. D – Do you need a tourniquet? If so, apply a tourniquet 2-3 inches above the injury. Twist, secure, and note the time applied. (TNCC pg. 220)

22. The key to safe and effective care of the trauma patient is associated with which of the following?
    a. Having multiple team leaders.
    b. Identified roles and responsibilities of the team members.
    c. Relying on conventional thinking.
    d. Engaging in individual goals for treatment.

B - Identified roles and responsibilities of the team members. Effective teams optimize resources and engage in a regular debriefing. (TNCC pg. 17)

PBD Nurse Education, LLC TCRN Posttest

1. Systemic vascular resistance (afterload) is decreased in which type of shock?
    a. Hypovolemic
    b. Cardiogenic
    c. Obstructive
    d. Distributive
2. Pulse pressure (PP) is widened in which disorder?
    a. Early shock.
    b. Increased intracranial pressure.
    c. Cardiac tamponade.
    d. Aortic valve stenosis.
3. A patient is diagnosed with a pelvic fracture and right tibial fracture after a motorcycle crash. Which classification of hypovolemic shock would most likely occur because of these injuries?
    a. Class I
    b. Class II
    c. Class III
    d. Class IV
4. A chest tube was just inserted on a patient with a tension pneumothorax. Which assessment finding would best indicate the treatment plan has been successful?
    a. Patient reports a decrease in chest pain.
    b. Presence of blood in the chest drainage system.
    c. Improved hemodynamic status.
    d. Decreased patient anxiety and diaphoresis.
5. Abdominal compartment syndrome is a form of which type of shock?
    a. Hypovolemic
    b. Cardiogenic
    c. Distributive
    d. Obstructive
6. A 20-year-old male was discharged home yesterday after a femur fracture from a fall. He returns today via EMS with dyspnea, tachypnea, and tachycardia. You notice a petechial rash over the axilla and peaked P waves on the EKG, so you suspect which disorder?
    a. Sepsis
    b. Disseminated Intravascular Coagulation (DIC)
    c. Fat emboli
    d. Rhabdomyolysis
7. A hazardous vulnerability assessment is completed in which emergency management phase?
    a. Mitigation
    b. Preparedness
    c. Response
    d. Recovery
8. Which is the best early indicator of shock in pediatric patients?
    a. Hypotension
    b. Tachypnea
    c. Decreased capillary refill.
    d. Tachycardia
9. Which type of skull fracture has the highest risk for developing an intracranial infection?
    a. Temporal bone fracture
    b. Depressed skull fracture
    c. Basilar skull fracture
    d. Linear skull fracture

10. A teenager dives into a shallow pool and completely transects his spinal cord. In addition to poikilothermia, which combination of assessment findings is commonly seen in neurogenic shock?
    a. Hypotension and bradycardia.
    b. Hypotension and tachycardia.
    c. Hypertension and bradycardia.
    d. Hypertension and tachycardia.
11. Advocating for bicycle lanes is an example of which phase of injury prevention?
    a. Primary
    b. Secondary
    c. Tertiary
    d. Quinary
12. The nurse is assessing a multi-trauma patient. Which of the following symptoms is an **EARLY** sign of shock?
    a. Restlessness
    b. Hypotension
    c. Bradycardia
    d. Weak peripheral pulses
13. The trauma nurse who works with community resources to distribute bike helmets and car seats is implementing which phase of injury prevention?
    a. Primary
    b. Secondary
    c. Tertiary
    d. Quinary
14. A 64-year-old patient with a history of atrial fibrillation fell yesterday hitting her head. She did not lose consciousness after the fall, but was found unresponsive this am. You suspect which type of brain hemorrhage?
    a. Epidural
    b. Subdural
    c. Subarachnoid
    d. Intracerebral
15. A 21-year-old male is brought in by EMS after a gunshot wound to the left flank while he was "running away from some dude." He can move his right leg but is unable to move his left leg. He has also lost pain and temperature sensation on the right side. You suspect:
    a. Anterior cord syndrome
    b. Brown-Sequard syndrome
    c. Central cord syndrome
    d. Posterior cord syndrome
16. A function of collecting data elements for trauma registry includes the following, **EXCEPT**:
    a. Evaluating clinical care.
    b. Developing injury prevention strategies.
    c. Assisting in staff debriefing.
    d. Verifying trauma center designation.
17. A 16-year-old male walks into the ED with a knife protruding from his abdomen. Your priority action is to:
    a. Remove the object and apply direct pressure.
    b. Stabilize the object.
    c. Initiate two large-bore IV's.
    d. Ordering an MRI to see where the knife blade is.

18. Which of the following statements in **INCORRECT** regarding trauma performance improvement (PI)?
    a. Trauma PI is multidisciplinary, and data driven.
    b. The PIPS plan pertains to the trauma center only, without feedback to referring facilities.
    c. Trauma PI fosters a culture of safety, transitioning from blame to opportunity.
    d. The key concepts are monitoring, evaluating, and improving performance.
19. Which symptom is considered the hallmark sign of compartment syndrome?
    a. Decreased distal pulses.
    b. Pulselessness.
    c. Pain out of proportion to the injury.
    d. No pain with movement of the affected extremity.
20. A patient presents to the ED after accidentally splashing lye in his eyes. Irrigation should continue until:
    a. The ocular pH reaches 7.4.
    b. Two liters of fluid has been instilled.
    c. The patient's visual acuity is 20/20.
    d. Blepharospasms decrease.
21. The following mechanisms of injury require transportation to a trauma center, **EXCEPT**:
    a. A fall two to three times the height of the child
    b. Motorcycle crash
    c. A fall > 20 feet in an adult
    d. Ejection from an automobile
22. Prior to calculating the total body surface area (TBSA), the recommended starting point for fluid resuscitation in an eight-year-old child with significant burn is:
    a. 125 mL/hour
    b. 250 mL/hour
    c. 375 mL/hour
    d. 500 mL/hour
23. Conditions or situations requiring a secured airway include the following, **EXCEPT**:
    a. Glasgow coma score (GCS) of 12 or less.
    b. Severe maxillofacial fractures.
    c. High risk of aspiration and the patient's inability to protect the airway.
    d. Inhalation injury with stridor and carbonaceous sputum.
24. A shift of the oxyhemoglobin dissociation curve to the right occurs in response to which of the following conditions?
    a. Hypothermia
    b. Carbon monoxide poisoning
    c. Methemoglobinemia
    d. Acidemia
25. The classic sign of this head injury is a transient loss of consciousness followed by a lucid period, and a second loss of consciousness.
    a. Subdural hematoma
    b. Intracerebral hematoma
    c. Epidural hematoma
    d. Diffuse axonal injury
26. Which incomplete spinal cord syndrome is characterized by loss of motor and sensory function in the upper extremities that is greater than that of the lower extremities?
    a. Central cord
    b. Brown-Sequard
    c. Anterior cord

d. Posterior cord

27. Mortality is the highest with injuries to which zone in the neck?
    a. Zone I
    b. Zone II
    c. Zone III
    d. Zone IV
28. Lip laceration or fractured teeth are commonly associated with which maxillary fracture?
    a. Le Fort I
    b. Le Fort II
    c. Le Fort III
    d. Le Fort IV
29. Laboratory indicators of rhabdomyolysis include the following, **EXCEPT**:
    a. Increased creatine kinase (CK) levels
    b. Myoglobinuria
    c. Elevation of aspartate aminotransferase (AST) levels
    d. Hypokalemia
30. Appropriate fluid resuscitation of the pediatric patient in hemorrhagic shock includes:
    a. Packed red blood cells administered as a bolus of 20 mL/kg.
    b. Infusion of 10 mL/kg of isotonic crystalloid solution over 20 minutes.
    c. Rapid infusion of 20 mL/kg of warmed isotonic crystalloid solution over 5-10 minutes.
    d. Blood product transfusion at a 1:1:2 ratio.
31. The normal range for fetal heart rate is between:
    a. 60-100 beats per minute.
    b. 100-150 beats per minute.
    c. 120-160 beats per minute.
    d. 150-200 beats per minute.
32. These medications can prevent the increase in heart rate that is an expected response in patients with hypovolemia and/or shock states.
    a. Positive inotropes
    b. Vasopressors
    c. ACE inhibiters
    d. Beta-blockers
33. Which of the following is the antidote for cyanide toxicity?
    a. 100% oxygen
    b. Hydroxocobalamin
    c. 2-PAM
    d. Atropine
34. The initial symptoms of acute radiation poisoning include:
    a. Nausea, vomiting, and diarrhea.
    b. Dyspnea and cherry red skin.
    c. Salivation and lacrimation.
    d. Cough, burning, and blisters.
35. In Simple Triage and Rapid Treatment (START) triage patients are sorted in a manner to allow the nurse to provide the most good to the greatest number of patients. The "walking wounded" are classified as:
    a. Black
    b. Red
    c. Yellow
    d. Green

36. Laboratory findings in disseminated intravascular coagulation (DIC) include:
    a. Elevated D-dimer and increased fibrinogen.
    b. Elevated fibrin degradation products and decreased fibrinogen.
    c. Prolonged PTT and increased platelet count.
    d. Decreased platelet count and increased fibrinogen.
37. What is a normal ankle-brachial index?
    a. 1.2-1.6
    b. 0.9-1.2
    c. 0.4-0.9
    d. < 0.4
38. What is a normal shock index?
    a. 0.5-.07
    b. 0.7-0.9
    c. 0.9-1.2
    d. 1.2-1.6
39. Diagnostic criteria for acute respiratory distress syndrome (ARDS) includes:
    a. Hypoxemia resolved by higher levels of oxygen.
    b. Clinical evidence of left ventricular failure.
    c. Partial pressure of oxygen/fraction of inspired oxygen ratio of less than 200 mm Hg.
    d. High pulmonary artery occlusive pressure.
40. Which of the following is a possible cause of hypercarbia ($ETCO_2 > 45$ mm Hg)?
    a. Increase in respiratory rate.
    b. Rapid rise in body temperature.
    c. Increase in tidal volume.
    d. Decrease in metabolic rate.
41. In drug-assisted intubation, which induction agent is preferred in trauma because it does not affect hemodynamic stability?
    a. Propofol
    b. Midazolam
    c. Etomidate
    d. Fentanyl
42. Which of the following physical findings may indicate globe rupture?
    a. Flashes of light and floaters in the visual field
    b. A teardrop-shaped pupil and vitreous humor leakage
    c. Halos around lights and tunnel vision
    d. Painless loss of vision and transient episodes of blindness
43. The treatment plan for hydrofluoric acid exposure includes which medication:
    a. Silvadene
    b. Polyethylene glycol (PEG)
    c. Calcium gluconate
    d. Sodium bicarbonate
44. Treatment for rib fractures includes the following, **EXCEPT**:
    a. Early mobilization to enhance chest wall expansion.
    b. Lidocaine(xylocaine) patches to reduce pain.
    c. Intercostal nerve blocks to reduce pain.
    d. Rib binding to support the chest wall.

45. Application of a pelvic binder is performed in unstable pelvic fractures to:
    a. Reduce muscle spasms.
    b. Prevent fat embolism.
    c. Temporarily tamponade the bleeding.
    d. Prevent compartment syndrome.
46. Appropriate management of an amputated finger includes storing it in which of the following?
    a. Distilled water
    b. Iodine gauze
    c. Saline-moistened gauze
    d. Ice water
47. A nonporous dressing is placed over an open chest wound to the right chest from a stab wound. Which finding indicates the treatment is ineffective?
    a. Decreasing oxygen saturation and tracheal shift to the left side.
    b. Chest wall pain.
    c. Respiratory rate remains at 32 breaths/minute.
    d. Flat jugular veins.
48. Hypotension in tension pneumothorax is the result of:
    a. Impaired venous return to the heart.
    b. Negative intrathoracic pressure.
    c. Vasodilation from distributive shock.
    d. Hemorrhage from the internal mammary artery.
49. Which injury is NOT typically seen from lap belt only restraint in an MVC?
    a. Small bowel rupture
    b. Renal injury
    c. Stomach rupture
    d. Chance fracture
50. Following a mass casualty event, a critical incident stress debriefing (CISD) is offered for the hospital staff who were directly involved in the care of the patients. The primary goal of holding a CISM is:
    a. Collecting information to prepare a media statement.
    b. Mitigating the impact of traumatic events and restoring adaptive functioning to those exposed.
    c. Identifying the staff who will require mental health counseling.
    d. Gaining information on the cause of the event to assist law enforcement.
51. What energy force results in tearing of the Achilles tendon?
    a. Compression
    b. Tension
    c. Shearing
    d. Torsion
52. Several impacts may occur during the evolution of a motor vehicle collision (MVC). Which impact may result in shearing the ligamentum arteriosus?
    a. First impact
    b. Second impact
    c. Third impact
    d. Forth impact
53. Quaternary blast injury produces which type of injury?
    a. Globe rupture
    b. Fragmentation injury
    c. Traumatic amputations
    d. Burns

54. Drug-assisted intubation (DAI) is performed to decrease the risk of aspiration and increase the chance of a successful emergent intubation. Which of the following medications used for paralysis is a depolarizing agent that stimulates cholinergic receptors?
    a. Succinylcholine (Anectine)
    b. Rocuronium (Zemuron)
    c. Vecuronium (Norcuron)
    d. Pancuronium (Pavulon)
55. Which of the following is an early finding in the patient with increased intracranial pressure (ICP)?
    a. Vomiting.
    b. Motor posturing.
    c. Widened pulse pressure.
    d. Reflex bradycardia.
56. Which brain injury follows a fracture of the temporal or parietal bone, lacerating the middle meningeal artery?
    a. Subdural hematoma
    b. Epidural hematoma
    c. Basilar skull fracture
    d. Intracerebral hematoma
57. A patient has a fractured sternum and chest to mid-scapular back pain from a high-speed motor vehicle collision (MVC.) Which radiologic finding in seen in aortic disruption?
    a. Blunting of the costophrenic angle.
    b. Enlarged cardiac silhouette.
    c. Mediastinum widening
    d. Pleural thickening
58. Axis (C2) fractures typically occur from which mechanism of injury?
    a. Hyperflexion
    b. Hyperextension
    c. Rotational
    d. Axial loading
59. Chance fractures predictably occur from which mechanism of injury?
    a. Hyperflexion
    b. Hyperextension
    c. Rotational
    d. Axial loading
60. Fracturing the ulnar shaft and dislocating the radial head while falling onto outstretched hands is referred to as which injury?
    a. Colles
    b. Scaphoid
    c. Monteggia's
    d. Galeazzi's

TCRN Posttest Answers

1. **D** – Afterload (systemic vascular resistance) is decreased in distributive shock due to vasodilation and maldistribution of blood. (TNCC pg. 97)
2. **B** – Pulse pressure is widened in increased intracranial pressure, one symptom of Cushing's response, along with bradycardia and decreased respiration. Pulse pressure is narrow in early shock. (TNCC pg. 116)
3. **D** – Pelvic fractures cause massive blood loss resulting in severe shock. (TNCC pg. 96)
4. **C** – The treatment is effective if the patient's vital signs (hemodynamics) improve. (TNCC pg. 155)
5. **D** – Abdominal compartment syndrome causes obstructive shock, along with cardiac tamponade and tension pneumothorax. (TNCC pg. 97)
6. **C** – The classic triad of symptoms of fat embolism is axillary petechial rash, along with sudden onset of restlessness and severe hypoxia. (TNCC pg. 442)

7. **A** – Completing a hazardous vulnerability assessment is completed during the mitigation phase of disaster management. (TNCC pg. 94)
8. **D** – Tachycardia and delayed capillary refill are early signs of poor tissue perfusion in the pediatric patient. (TNCC pg. 277)
9. **C** – A complication of basilar skull fractures is infection so do not pack ears or nose. (TNCC pg. 131)
10. **A** – The loss of sympathetic nervous system stimulation and unopposed parasympathetic stimulation results in bradycardia and hypotension in neurogenic shock. (TNCC pg. 97)
11. **A** – Primary prevention is focused on preventing the occurrence of the injury, so advocating for bicycle lanes is primary prevention. (TNCC pg. 4)
12. **A** – Restlessness, anxiety, tachycardia, and narrowed pulse pressure are seen in early shock. (TNCC pg. 92)
13. **B** – Secondary prevention focuses on reducing the severity of the injury, and distributing car seats reduces the severity of injury in an MVC. (TNCC pg. 4)
14. **B** – Subdural bleeds result from tearing of the bridging veins resulting in a steady decline in level of consciousness. (TNCC pgs. 127-128)
15. **B** – Brown-Sequard results in ipsilateral motor loss and contralateral loss of pain sensation, typically seen in penetrating injury. (TNCC pg. 202)
16. **C** – The purpose of collecting data for trauma registry is to design prevention strategies and improve care. (*American College of Surgeons Optimal Care of the Injured Patient.*)
17. **B** – Stabilize impaled objects to tamponade bleeding. (TNCC pg. 130)
18. **B** – Performance improvement is a system of multidisciplinary reviews with a feedback loop to identify areas for improvement and develop an action plan. (TNCC pg. 20)
19. **C** – Pain out of proportion to the injury is the classic sign of compartment syndrome. Keep the extremity in neutral position and do not apply ice. (TNCC pg. 209)
20. **A** – Lye is an alkaline substance (pH 14) so irrigation should continue until the ocular pH reaches 7.4. (TNCC pgs. 132-134)
21. **B** – Motorcycle crashes at > 20 mph meet criteria for transporting to a trauma center, not all motorcycle crashes. (TNCC pg. 31)
22. **B** – The recommended starting points for fluid resuscitation rates prior to burn calculation are 250 mL/hour for ages 6-13 years of age, 125 mL/hour for 5 years of age and younger, and 500 mL/hour for 14 years and older. (TNCC pg. 239)
23. **A** – A Glasgow coma score (GCS) of 8 or less requires a secured airway. (TNCC pg. 46)
24. **D** – Acidemia (decreased pH), increased carbon dioxide (hypercapnia), and hyperthermia shift the oxyhemoglobin curve to the right, so oxygen is released to the tissues. (TNCC pgs. 75-76)
25. **C** – The classic signs/symptoms of an epidural hematoma is loss of consciousness, lucid period with second loss of consciousness. Additional symptoms include ipsilateral pupil dilation and contralateral hemiparesis. (TNCC pg. 127)
26. **A** – Central cord syndrome most frequently occurs due to hyperextension, in older adults. (TNCC pg. 202)
27. **A** – Mortality is the highest with injuries to zone I in the neck where major vessels and trachea are located. Symptoms include dysphonia, dysphagia, and subcutaneous emphysema. (TNCC pgs. 143-144)
28. **A** – Assessment findings seen in a transverse maxillary bone fracture (Le Fort) include lip laceration or fractured teeth and malocclusion. (TNCC pgs. 131-132)
29. **D** – Laboratory indicators of rhabdomyolysis include an elevated CK, myoglobin, and potassium. Signs/symptoms of rhabdomyolysis include muscle pain and dark red urine. (TNCC pg. 447)
30. **C** – Interventions include rapid infusion of 20 mL/kg of warmed isotonic crystalloid solution (NS or LR) over 5-10 minutes with a three-way stopcock and a 20-mL syringe. Blood products are administered at 10 mL/kg. (TNCC pg. 278)
31. **C** – The normal fetal heart rate is 120-160 beats per minute and may be heard using a Doppler ultrasound at 10 weeks gestation. (TNCC pg. 334)

32. **D** – Beta blockers may mask tachycardia, an early sign of shock. (TNCC pg. 324)
33. **B** – Hydroxocobalamin is the antidote for cyanide toxicity, turns urine red. Oxygen is the antidote for carbon monoxide toxicity. Atropine at 2-PAM are the antidotes for nerve agent exposure like Sarin gas and VX, and organophosphates. (Sheehy pg. 413)
34. **A** – Symptoms of acute radiation syndrome begin with nausea, vomiting, headache, and diarrhea. Radiation exposure may be from a "dirty bomb". Salivation and lacrimation are seen in nerve agent exposure. (TNCC pg. 422)
35. **D** – The "walking wounded" are classified using the green triage tag color. Red is immediate, yellow is delayed, green is minor, and black is unlikely to survive. (TNCC pg. 409)
36. **B** – Laboratory findings in DIC include elevated fibrin degradation products and D-dimer, prolonged PT and PTT, and decreased platelet count and fibrinogen. (TNCC pg. 445)
37. **B** – Normal ankle-brachial index (ABI) is 0.9-1.2 and is used to detect peripheral vascular injuries. 0.4-0.9 indicates moderate peripheral arterial disease, and < 0.4 indicates severe occlusion or disease. (Sheehy pg. 136)
38. **A** – Shock index is heart rate (HR) divided by systolic blood pressure (SBP) Normal shock index is 0.5-0.7. The higher the number, the poorer the outcome. EX: 80/120 = .67.
39. **C** – P:F ratio of < 200 mm Hg is diagnostic for ARDS, along with normal PA pressures, and refractory hypoxemia. P:F ratios of 201-300 mm Hg is diagnostic for acute lung injury (ALI), ideal P:F ratio is > 400 mm Hg. (TNCC pgs. 442-443)
40. **B** – Possible causes of hypercarbia include a rapid rise in body temperature (suspect infection), increase in metabolic rate, and a decrease in respiratory rate (retaining CO_2). (TNCC pg. 438)
41. **C** – Etomidate has minimal effects on hemodynamic stability. Midazolam, Fentanyl, and Propofol decrease mean arterial pressure (MAP). (TNCC pg. 85)
42. **B**- A teardrop-shaped pupil and vitreous humor leakage is indicative of globe rupture. (TNCC pgs. 132-134)
43. **C** – Calcium gluconate is used for hydrofluoric acid (used for glass etching) burns since fluoride binds with calcium in the blood. (TNCC pg. 247)
44. **D** – Binding ribs may push a jagged edge into the lungs causing a pneumothorax, so not recommended. pg. 439
45. **C** – Pelvic binder application will help attain stabilization and control hemorrhage by exerting external pressure. (TNCC pg. 178)
46. **C** – Keep the amputated finger cool by wrapping it in saline-moistened sterile gauze, and then place it in a sealed plastic bag. Place that bag on top of a second bag of ice. Do not freeze the amputated part by putting it in the ice water. (TNCC pg. 217)
47. **A** – Decreased oxygen saturation and tracheal shift to the unaffected side indicates tension pneumothorax so remove the dressing and reevaluate the patient. (TNCC pg. 147)
48. **A** – Air enters the pleural space but cannot escape on expiration, increasing intrathoracic pressure. As pressure rises, venous return is impaired, cardiac output decreases, and hypotension occurs. (TNCC pg. 147)
49. **B** – Lap belt only restraint may cause hollow organ (bowel and stomach) injury and/or a chance fracture of T12-L2 from hyperflexion. (TNCC pg. 171)
50. **B** – Critical Incident Stress Debriefing (CISD) promotes communication and promotes resiliency. Those affected by the event are invited, but not forced to participate. (Sheehy pg. 25)
51. **B** – Tension forces stretch tendons by tugging on the ends. (TNCC pg. 27)
52. **C** – In the third impact, internal structures collide within the body cavity. (TNCC pg. 28)
53. **D** – Quaternary blast injury causes burns. Primary injury causes globe rupture and rupturing tympanic membranes. The secondary impact injuries are from projectiles. Tertiary injuries such as amputations are due to propulsion. Hazardous material exposure is quinary blast injury. (TNCC pg. 35)
54. **A** – Succinylcholine is a depolarizing agent that is a known trigger of malignant hyperthermia. Symptoms of malignant hyperthermia include high fever, increased CO_2, muscle rigidity, and metabolic acidosis. Treatment includes rapid cooling and Dantrolene. (TNCC pg. 85)

55. **A** – Vomiting, headache, and restlessness are early symptoms of increased ICP. Abnormal motor posturing, dilated nonresponsive pupils, unresponsiveness, and Cushing's triad of widened pulse pressure, bradycardia, and altered respiratory pattern are late symptoms of increased intracranial pressure. (Sheehy pg. 191)
56. **B** – Epidural hematomas (EDH) are frequently associated with fractures of the temporal or parietal bones that lacerate the middle meningeal artery. Classic symptoms of EDH include a transient loss of consciousness, followed by a period of lucidity, with a secondary loss of consciousness. (TNCC pg. 129)
57. **C** – Mediastinum widening, obscured aortic knob, and an apical cap are the most common radiologic findings seen in aortic disruption. Blunting of the costophrenic angle is seen in pleural effusion. An enlarged cardiac silhouette is seen in pericardial tamponade. (TNCC pg. 158)
58. **B** – Axis (C2) vertebral neck fractures are caused by hyperextension. Atlanto-occipital (C1) vertebral neck fractures are due to hyperflexion. (TNCC pg. 204)
59. **A** – Hyperflexion causes Chance lumbar (seat belt) fractures. Suspect concurrent hollow organ abdominal injuries. (TNCC pg. 205)
60. **C** – Monteggia's fracture is an ulnar shaft fracture with radial head dislocation. A Colles fracture is a distal radius fracture. A scaphoid fracture is a break of one of the small bones of the hand. Galeazzi's fracture is a distal radial fracture with a distal ulnar epiphyseal fracture. (TNCC pg. 197)

PDB Nurse Education TCRN "Critical Thinking"

1. Is the Trauma Medical Director required to hold a current Advanced Trauma Life Support (**ATLS**) certification?
2. Is the Trauma Program Manager position required to have 1.0 full-time equivalent (**FTE**) commitment to the trauma program?
3. Are all trauma centers required to have an **injury prevention** program?
4. What is the required patient-to-nurse ratio in the ICU in all trauma centers?
5. Is an emergency physician's discretion one of the eight criteria for a full trauma activation?
6. What is the maximum hours of **trauma diversion** for a trauma center during that reporting period?
7. What GCS is considered a severe traumatic brain injury (TBI) with head CT evidence of intracranial trauma?
8. Which level trauma center is expected to provide **initial definitive care** of all injuries?
9. What is the purpose of "**just culture**"?
10. Lung barotrauma occurs from which **blast** pressure?
11. How would you triage a stable patient with an eyelid laceration utilizing the Emergency Severity Index (**ESI**) triage?
12. **Sacral sparing** in conjunction with focal deficits is associated with which spinal cord injuries (SCI)?
13. What color does a **colorimetric CO_2** detector turn in the presence of carbon dioxide?
14. Why do you administer a **sedative** prior to a paralytic in drug-assisted intubation?
15. Why do you auscultate over the epigastrium prior to listening for bilateral breath sounds after endotracheal intubation?
16. Decreased 2,3 DPG from transfusing banked blood shifts the oxyhemoglobin dissociation curve in which direction?
17. Cardiac output (CO) is heart rate (HR) times stroke volume (SV). Stroke volume is dependent on Preload, afterload, and contractility. How does hemorrhagic shock affect preload?
18. How does the release of aldosterone help the body compensate for shock?
19. A patient with a femur fracture has a heart rate of 130 bpm with a systolic blood pressure of 70 mm Hg. Which class of hemorrhagic shock do these vital signs reflect?
20. Which shock occurs due to the loss of sympathetic nervous system control of vascular tone?
21. Why is **hypocalcemia** a risk when transfusing banked blood?

22. What is the purpose of viscoelastic (**TEG**, TEM, ROTEM) testing?
23. How do you calculate cerebral perfusion pressure (**CPP**)?
24. What are the four components of FOUR (**F**ull **O**utline of **U**n**R**esponsiveness) score?
25. Which cranial nerves are assessed when evaluating extraocular movements (**EOM's**)?
26. What is normal **intraocular pressure**?
27. What is **pulsus paradoxus**?
28. What are common musculoskeletal injuries seen with falls onto outstretched hands (**FOOSH**)?
29. What two clinical decision tools does TNCC teach to assess the need for **cervical spine** imaging following trauma?
30. What is the initial treatment of **frostbite** in the emergency department?
31. Why is shaving hair around the laceration contraindicated in repair?
32. What fluid is used in burn fluid resuscitation?
33. What is the recommended formula for calculating fluid replacement for an adult with > 20% thermal burn after TBSA has been determined?
34. Why are calcium levels monitored in **hydrofluoric acid** exposure?
35. What is **trans broken arm** syndrome?
36. How is "**TEN-4 FACES P**" useful in remembering suspicious bruising?
37. How is untreated **sleep apnea** related to trauma?
38. What is the **SPICES** mnemonic for assessing frailty risk?
39. What is **supine hypotension syndrome**?
40. What acid base imbalance is a normal finding in advanced pregnancy?
41. Utilizing **START** triage, the walking wounded are classified with which tag?
42. What is the initial management for Sarin gas exposure?
43. When do most **fat emboli** occur after long bone fracture?
44. What is the treatment plan for acute lung injury (ALI) and acute respiratory distress syndrome (**ARDS**)?
45. What are the components of the **ABCEF** Bundle to prevent post-operative complications?
46. Which medical conditions increase the risk of intra-abdominal hypertension (IAH)?
47. Why is continuous cardiac monitoring required for patients diagnosed with rhabdomyolysis?
48. What is the goal urine output in the management of rhabdomyolysis?
49. At what age does the American College of Surgeons (ACS) require screening for **alcohol misuse**?
50. What is Hamman's sign?
51. How can the "lethal triad" of trauma be avoided?
52. What are key points to teach the caregivers of a child with a **hip spica cast**?
53. Wearing chest protection while playing contact sports and ensuring automatic external defibrillators (AEDs) are available at sporting events can decrease the risk of sudden cardiac arrest from what type of blunt cardiac injury?
54. Why is it important to document a child's weight in **kilograms** only?
55. Where do you assess **capillary refill** in children?
56. What memory tool is useful to remember **hypotension** in children ages 1-10?
57. How would you explain procedural **sedation** to a child?
58. Why do you NOT wrap a tibial intraosseous (**IO**) needle circumferentially?
59. How do you treat the pain of fluid administration through an intraosseous (**IO**) needle?
60. Why are **rib fractures** a red flag for child maltreatment?
61. What **burns** are more suspicious for child maltreatment?
62. Are pediatric trauma centers required to have a child life specialist?
63. Difficulty **swallowing** occurs after injury to which cranial nerve?
64. Why is asking "What happened to you?" better than asking "What is wrong with you?"
65. What is "**the pause**?"

66. Who is responsible for ensuring qualified transport personnel accompany the patient to a specialized pediatric center?
67. A roofer who fell 20 feet is transported to your local emergency department. A **CT scan** of the spine is ordered since the patient is unable to move his lower extremities. Does EMTALA require a CT scan prior to transporting the patient to a trauma center?
68. What are the components of **Virchow's triad** that leads to venous thrombosis?
69. How does a massive **pulmonary embolus** (PE) affect the heart?
70. How can **ventilator-associated pneumonia** (VAP) be prevented?

TCRN "Critical Thinking" Answers

1. Is the Trauma Medical Director required to hold a current Advanced Trauma Life Support (**ATLS**) certification? Yes. (ACS pg. 16)
2. Is the Trauma Program Manager position required to have 1.0 full-time equivalent (**FTE**) commitment to the trauma program? Yes. (ACS pg. 18)
3. Are all trauma centers required to have an **injury prevention** program? Yes, examples include child passenger safety seat education, bicycle safety/helmet initiatives, fall prevention, and Stop the Bleed programs. (ACS pg. 20)
4. What is the required patient-to-nurse ratio in the **ICU** in all trauma centers? The patient-to-nurse ratio in the ICU must be 1:1 or 2:1 depending on patient acuity. (ACS pg. 60)
5. Is an emergency physician's discretion one of the eight criteria for a full trauma activation? Yes. (ACS pg. 81)
6. What are the maximum hours of **trauma diversion** for a trauma center during that reporting period? Trauma centers must not exceed 400 hours of diversion during the reporting period. (ACS pg. 94)
7. What GCS is considered a severe traumatic brain injury (**TBI**) with head CT evidence of intracranial trauma? A severe TBI is considered a **GCS < 9** with head CT evidence of intracranial trauma. (ACS pg. 95)
8. Which level trauma center is expected to provide **initial definitive care** of all injuries? Level II trauma centers are not expected to provide comprehensive care, just initial definite care. (TNCC pgs. 15 & 426)
9. What is the purpose of "**just culture**"? No repercussion for reporting near misses and errors enables accurate root cause analysis and identification of the system issues that contribute to errors. (TNCC pg. 21)
10. Lung barotrauma occurs from which **blast** pressure? Primary injury such as "blast lung" occurs from pressure. (TNCC pg. 35)
11. How would you triage a stable patient with an eyelid laceration utilizing the Emergency Severity Index (ESI) triage? **ESI triage** level 3 with two expected resources, specialty consultation and laceration repair/ (TNCC pg. 52 and ESI Triage)
12. **Sacral sparing** in conjunction with focal deficits is associated with which spinal cord injuries (SCI)? Patients with incomplete spinal cord injuries retain anal sphincter tone. (TNCC pg. 55)
13. What color does a **colorimetric CO_2** detector turn in the presence of carbon dioxide? Yellow when the CO_2 is > 15 mm Hg, verifying endotracheal (ETT) intubation. (TNCC pg. 67)
14. Why do you administer a **sedative** prior to a paralytic in drug-assisted intubation? The patient may experience pain, resulting in tachycardia and increased intracranial pressure. (TNCC pg. 74)
15. Why do you **auscultate** over the epigastrium prior to listening for bilateral breath sounds after endotracheal intubation? Auscultate over the epigastrium first since positive-pressure ventilation causes gastric distension and increases the risk of aspiration. (TNCC pgs. 69 and 75)
16. Decreased 2,3 DPG from transfusing banked blood shifts the **oxyhemoglobin** dissociation curve in which direction? The curve shifts to the left and hemoglobin holds onto oxygen. (TNCC pg. 76)
17. Cardiac output (CO) is heart rate (HR) times stroke volume (SV). Stroke volume is dependent on Preload, afterload, and contractility. How does hemorrhagic shock affect **preload**? Preload (end-diastolic volume) is decreased in hemorrhagic shock. (TNCC pgs. 90 and 142)

18. How does the release of **aldosterone** help the body compensate for shock? Aldosterone release increases reabsorption of sodium and water, increasing intravascular volume. (TNCC pg. 94)
19. A patient with a femur fracture has a heart rate of 130 bpm with a systolic blood pressure of 70 mm Hg. Which **class of hemorrhagic** shock do these vital signs reflect? Class III (moderate). (TNCC pg. 96)
20. Which shock occurs due to the loss of sympathetic nervous system control of vascular tone? **Neurogenic** shock is seen in spinal cord injury, unopposed parasympathetic activity results in bradycardia. (TNCC pgs. 97-98)
21. Why is **hypocalcemia** a risk when transfusing banked blood? Citrate chelates calcium, rendering it inactive, permitting continued bleeding. Treat with calcium gluconate or calcium chloride. (TNCC pg. 99)
22. What is the purpose of viscoelastic (**TEG**, TEM, ROTEM) testing? Viscoelastic testing evaluates platelet function, clot strength, and fibrinolysis. (TNCC pgs. 104-105)
23. How do you calculate cerebral perfusion pressure (**CPP**)? Cerebral perfusion pressure (CPP) = mean arterial pressure (MAP) – intracranial pressure (ICP). Normal CPP = 60-80 mmHg. (TNCC pg. 116)
24. What are the four components of FOUR (**F**ull **O**utline of **U**n**R**esponsiveness) score? Eye response, motor response, brainstem reflexes, respiration. (TNCC pgs. 120-123)
25. Which cranial nerves are assessed when evaluating extraocular movements (**EOM's**)? Cranial nerves III, IV, and VI. (TNCC pg. 125)
26. What is normal **intraocular pressure**? Normal pressure readings are 10-21 mmHg. (TNCC pg. 128)
27. What is **pulsus paradoxus**? A drop in systolic blood pressure of 10 mm Hg or more during inspiration. (TNCC pg. 158)
28. What are common musculoskeletal injuries seen with falls onto outstretched hands (**FOOSH**)? Colles, Scaphoid, Monteggia's, and Galeazzi fractures. (TNCC pgs. 196-197)
29. What two clinical decision tools does TNCC teach to assess the need for **cervical spine** imaging following trauma? Canadian C-Spine Rule and NEXUS. Which tool does your facility utilize? (TNCC pgs. 213, 224, 225)
30. What is the initial treatment of **frostbite** in the emergency department? Gently rewarm in water between 40 and 42 degrees Celsius for 15 to 30 minutes and provide adequate pain control. (TNCC pg. 233)
31. Why is **shaving** hair around the laceration contraindicated in repair. Shaving hair increases the risk of infection. (TNCC pg. 234)
32. What fluid is used in burn fluid resuscitation? **Lactated Ringer's** solution, not abnormal saline. (TNCC pgs. 239-240)
33. What is the recommended formula for calculating fluid replacement for an adult with > 20% thermal burn after TBSA has been determined? **LR at 2 mL/kg times the percentage of TBSA**. Half of the fluid is infused in the first 8 hours from the time of the burn injury. (TNCC pgs. 239-240)
34. Why are calcium levels monitored in **hydrofluoric acid** exposure? Hydrofluoric acid depletes calcium levels. (TNCC pg. 247)
35. What is **trans broken arm** syndrome? Focusing on gender or genitalia instead of the presenting issue. (TNCC pg. 261)
36. How is "**TEN-4 FACES P**" useful in remembering suspicious bruising? Bruising to the **T**orso, **E**ars, or **N**eck in children under 4 years of age. Bruising to the **F**renulum, **A**ngle of jaw/ear, **C**heek, **E**yelid, **S**ubconjunctiva, and **P**atterned injuries. (TNCC pg. 285)
37. How is untreated **sleep apnea** related to trauma? Drivers with untreated sleep apnea are often drowsy while driving, translating to a 243% higher risk for MVC. (TNCC pg. 299)
38. What is the SPICES mnemonic for assessing frailty risk? **S**kin integrity, **P**roblems eating, **I**ncontinence, **C**onfusion, **E**vidence of falls, **S**leep disturbance. (TNCC pg. 327)
39. What is **supine hypotension syndrome**? Aortocaval compression from a gravid uterus when the patient is supine. (TNCC pg. 333)
40. What acid base imbalance is a normal finding in advanced **pregnancy**? Respiratory alkalosis occurs since pregnant patients breathe faster, blowing off carbon dioxide. (TNCC pg. 334)

41. Utilizing **START** triage, the walking wounded are classified with which tag? Green for minor care. (TNCC pg. 409)
42. What is the initial management for **Sarin gas** exposure? Don your PPE, decontaminate the patient, administer atropine and 2-PAM. (TNCC pg. 418)
43. When do most **fat emboli** occur after long bone fracture? Most fat emboli occur within 24-72 hours after long bone fracture. (TNCC pg. 442)
44. What is the treatment plan for acute lung injury (ALI) and acute respiratory distress syndrome (**ARDS**)? Lower tidal volumes, PEEP between 10- and 15-mm Hg, prone positioning, high-frequency ventilation, and extracorporeal membrane oxygenation (ECMO). (TNCC pg. 443)
45. What are the components of the **ABCEF** Bundle to prevent post-operative complications? **A** is for **a**ssessing, preventing, and managing pain. **B** is for **b**oth spontaneous awakening trials and spontaneous breathing trials. **C** is for the **c**hoice of analgesia and sedation. **D** is assessing, preventing, and managing **d**elirium. **E** is for **e**xercise and **e**arly mobilization. **F** is for **f**amily engagement and empowerment. (TNCC pgs. 443-444)
46. Which medical conditions increase the risk of intra-abdominal hypertension (**IAH**)? Patients who are morbidly obese, have chronic ascites, or are pregnant. (TNCC pg. 446)
47. Why is continuous cardiac monitoring required for patients diagnosed with rhabdomyolysis? **Hyperkalemia** leads to cardiac irritability, so ECG monitoring is required. (TNCC pg. 447)
48. What is the goal of **urine output** in the management of rhabdomyolysis? Urine output of 100-300 mL/hour. Alkalinization of urine may promote diuresis. (TNCC pg. 447)
49. At what age does the American College of Surgeons (ACS) require screening for **alcohol misuse**? The ACS requires trauma centers to screen all admitted trauma patients greater than 12 years old for alcohol misuse with a validated tool or routine blood alcohol content testing. (TNCC pg. 448)
50. What is **Hamman's** sign? Crunching sound synchronized with the heartbeat due to subcutaneous air. (Sheehy pg. 157)
51. How can the "**lethal triad**" of trauma be avoided? Keep the patient warm, provide early hemorrhage control, and avoid excessive crystalloid administration. (Sheehy pg. 166)
52. What are key points to teach the caregivers of a child with a **hip spica cast**? The child will be in the cast for 4 to 12 weeks, so avoid getting it wet. Monitor the skin closely for pressure points. You will need a special car seat.
53. Wearing chest protection while playing contact sports and ensuring automatic external defibrillators (AEDs) are available at sporting events can decrease the risk of sudden cardiac arrest from what type of blunt cardiac injury? **Commotio cordis** results in ventricular fibrillation. (Sheehy pg. 156)
54. Why is it important to document a child's **weight in kilograms (kg)** only? Pediatric medication dosing is based on kilograms, and double dosing may be lethal. (ENPC pgs. 33 and 60)
55. Where do you assess **capillary refill** in children? Blanch the forehead, sole of foot, or palm of hand. Normal capillary refill is 2 seconds or less. (TNCC pg. 277)
56. What memory tool is useful to remember **hypotension** in children ages 1-10? Systolic blood pressure (SBP) < 70 + (2 x age in years). (TNCC pg. 277)
57. How would you explain **procedural sedation** to a child? "Take a nap." not "Put you to sleep."
58. Why do you NOT wrap a **tibial intraosseous** (IO) needle circumferentially? An early sign of IO infiltration is swelling behind the site, and it is easily missed if the site is covered. (ENPC pg. 37)
59. How do you treat the **pain** of fluid administration through an intraosseous (IO) needle? Plain xylocaine.
60. Why are rib fractures a **red flag** for child maltreatment? Infant cartilage is bendable and more difficult to break. (ENPC pg. 36)
61. What burns are more suspicious for **child maltreatment**? Clearly demarcated burns of the lower legs to feet (sock-like), hands (glove-like), or buttocks (donut pattern) due to intentional dunking in scalding water, or patterned burns from an iron or cigarette. (ENPC pg. 133)
62. Are pediatric trauma centers required to have a child life specialist? Yes. (ACS pg. 24)

63. Difficulty swallowing occurs after injury to which cranial nerve? **CN IX**, glossopharyngeal. (Sheehy pg. 176)
64. Why is asking "What happened to you?" better than asking "What is wrong with you?" It follows **trauma-informed care** approach avoiding retraumatization. (ENPC pg. 270)
65. What is "the pause?" A period of silence after a patient's death to **honor** their life. It highlights the human aspect of healthcare, fostering staff well-being. (ENPC pg. 273)
66. Who is responsible for ensuring qualified transport personnel accompany the patient to a specialized pediatric center? The **transferring facility** arranges appropriate transport of the patient, in accordance with the provisions of EMTALA. (ENPC pg. 25)
67. A roofer who fell 20 feet is transported to your local emergency department. A CT scan of the spine is ordered since the patient is unable to move his lower extremities. Does EMTALA require a CT scan prior to transporting the patient to a trauma center? No, **do not delay** patient transfer. (TNCC pg. 104)
68. What are the components of **Virchow's triad** that leads to venous thrombosis? Stasis, endothelial damage, and hypercoagulopathy. The Caprini scale stratifies the risk of venous thrombosis in surgical patients. Symptoms include throbbing pain, leg swelling, and warm skin. (TNCC pgs. 440-441)
69. How does a massive **pulmonary embolus** (PE) affect the heart? A massive PE may cause **right heart failure**. Symptoms include abrupt pleuritic chest pain, apprehension, tachypnea, and tachycardia. (TNCC pg. 442)
70. How can **ventilator-associated pneumonia** (VAP) be prevented? Elevate the head of the bed 30-45 degrees, chlorhexidine oral care, and extubate as soon as medically possible. (TNCC pg. 443)

Made in the USA
Monee, IL
13 September 2026

62981962R00044